PRAISE FOR *BE THE BEST U*

"This is such an inspiring and uplifting book full of positives. It's these positives told with care and gentle humour, where there is no judgement, just a desire to help people live a better, more fulfilling life for themselves."

Amanda J Spedding – award-winning author
and graphic novelist

"Sharon is on a mission to help you feel better about yourself, your experiences, your abilities and to succeed in your life. With every inspiring word expressed in her warm, straight to the point style, Sharon supports her readers to see the value of embracing their uniqueness and the sum of everything they have experienced."

Julie Postance – author of *Breaking the Sound Barriers*

"This book is a refreshing reminder of the concepts and ideas we know (or may have forgotten) on how to take action so the real 'U' can emerge! There is no greater gift to ourselves than self acceptance and self love! Definitely worth a read."

Maggie – yoga teacher

THRIVE & SHINE CLIENTS

"Being a more mature client, a combination of Kinesiology and massage every fortnight to maintain my health, has worked for me over the past 15 years with Sharon. I leave her treatment room feeling strong, healthy, on top of the world and able to continue with my busy life."

Ula – client

"Like many others, I have struggled with family issues from a young age, which led me onto a very destructive path as I was holding on to so many painful memories. In 17 years of seeing a variety of other health professionals, no one has come close to the positive impact Sharon has had on my life. Treating the body, mind and spirit as a whole is her passion. I travel two hours for these sessions and over the past two years I have learnt to move forward and love myself again (a work in progress but I am getting there). I am now in a happier space and I recommend her Kinesiology/PSYCH-K® sessions to anybody who is struggling with their health, be it mental or physical. Thank you my health angel for your ongoing support."

Celeste – client

"I had severe restriction of movement in my left arm after tearing a muscle. I had several Kinesiology sessions with Sharon and I now have no pain and full movement in my arm. Kinesiology is also a great way to de-stress."

Sue – client

BE THE BEST U!

BY SHARON CAIRNS

Published in Australia by
Thrive and Shine Health
sharoncairnsrye@gmail.com
www.thriveandshinehealth.com.au

First published in Australia 2019
Second edition published in Australia 2025

National Library of Australia Cataloguing in Publication entry

A catalogue record for this
book is available from the
National Library of Australia

ISBN: 978-0-6486838-0-3 (paperback)
ISBN: 978-0-6486838-1-0 (epub)

Publishing Consultant Julie Postance www.iinspiremedia.com.au
Cover Design by 99 Designs
Layout and design by Sophie White Design www.sophiewhite.com.au
Editing by Pheonix Editing Amanda J. Spedding www.pheonixediting.com

Printed by Ingram Spark

DEDICATIONS

Special dedication to my dad, Peter, who died at 41 in a workplace accident. Thank you for being a health guru all those years ago and teaching me at a young age that the human body is such an amazing machine that has the ability to heal itself. I eventually followed your path!

To my three amazing Son's their partners and beautiful families - I am so blessed and proud to be your mum, mum-in-law and beach nanna. Thank you for all the love, joy, happiness, challenges, acceptance, patience and lessons in life that inspired me to write this book to support others - lets Celebrate!

I would like you to remember me as the Woman who always got back up!

My awesome and loving grandparents, Nanna and Pop; our special angel, Chloe, who throughout my life has been my aunty, sister, friend, and now they are all my guardian angels. Without you three in my life...

My book was revised and reprinted in 2025 due to major unexpected personal life changes. Starting again showed me more life lessons and a new layer of Being the Best Me! Now enjoying an even more positive, healthy, happy, balanced and peaceful life with many wonderful opportunities to Thrive and Shine which became my new business name!

Thank you to everyone who supported me - much love and gratitude.

♡

CONTENTS

INTRODUCTION

Being the Best U was written to inspire you with simple techniques and wisdom drawn from my life experiences, combined with my professional knowledge as a qualified Kinesiologist and Bioresonance Practitioner, guiding my clients to healthier, happier pathways to being their best. No one else's version of best but their own!

Anyone of any age who feels unsure about life and who they are, and who is looking for skills and direction to improve their life: this is for U!

You will be guided through this journal with life skills to support transforming U to your greatness, and understanding that it's ok to be U. So many life experiences hold us back from reaching our full potential, that stop us from moving forward. Learn about building your self-worth and confidence, to dump the past, dysfunction, and fear. To just let go to discover who U really are through love, respect, forgiveness and taking responsibility for *U!*

This will lead you on the pathway of better health, happiness, relationships, and balance in all areas of your life. We are only given one life, and we never know for how long. Why not learn to live your life well.

Challenge yourself to start right now!

Embrace, Enjoy, and Believe
in Being the Best U

MY OWN HEALTH STORY AND JOURNEY OF LEARNING

I have written this book to support others to believe they can change their life! I am passionate about making a difference.

This book has been designed as an easy read full of tips, knowledge and a bit of action. It is drawn from many years of life experience and supporting others as a natural health practitioner.

My story began as the eldest of six children born into a financially poor and dysfunctional family. There were happy times, but as the years went by, so did dysfunction, disruption, drama, and much insecurity. We didn't have much but wherever home was at the time, it was clean, there was always food on the table and clothes on our backs. As a family we struggled through unemployment, bushfires, ill health, moving homes and schools many, many times, mental health issues, death, drugs and suicide. Some of us survived but sadly there were a few casualties along the way. I will always be truly grateful that my grandparents, and parents who followed, later moved to this beautiful coastal area – a wonderful environment to live, work and raise a family.

There is no blame and I am not a victim – it was as it was!

Most families experience dysfunction, some just more than others. We all have our personal family-life stories. Just because they are family – either blood or by marriage – if they can't show respect to you as the person you are, it shows their lack of respect for themselves. They usually have a big hole within them that needs much healing. Whether they choose to accept this in their lifetime and make changes, is up to them. However, *never* let them drag you down to their level of unhappiness, insecurity, and lack of being able to love themselves and move forward.

We are either open and honest about our dysfunction and choose to change, get out of our comfort zone and grow or we can cover up the dysfunction and project to the world the perfect family. "What will people think?" is no way to move through the world, and it perpetuates the same dysfunctional cycle!

We are only human, after all. None of us are perfect, and that's ok but we always have a choice to make changes.

Good parenting is the biggest job in the world with no training, relying only on what we learnt (or didn't learn) from our parents. You do the best job you can with the knowledge you have at the time, and down the track, that knowledge can change. It's called hindsight.

My personal health life story has been the foundation for this book.

Being the eldest and 'second mum' to my five siblings, taught me a lot about both running a household and of motherhood. At the age of twelve, I was abducted and raped. The perpetrators were not family or friends but it was a secret that I kept even from my parents. I was threatened with a knife if I said a word about it, so most of my life I never felt safe. However, I never related the safety issue to the incident until I was a fair way into adulthood. Becoming a mum helped me through not feeling safe as I now had to provide a safe, stable home for my family. Periods of ill health, marriage, motherhood, self-education, working mum, deaths, divorce, single parenting, raising boys, relationship (second time around), step mum, blended families and now grandchildren, has been my life of growth.

During my early thirties, and being a mum to three small boys, I became extremely ill over some months; a slow decline in all areas of my health. I lost the coordination to use my left and right hands at the same time, unable to even cook my boys an egg due to the left and right side of my brain and my body not talking to each other. No energy, weight loss, and a lack of joy for life, my immune system was shot! I was emotionally devastated as I was unable to care properly for my boys or even drive a car; walking to the letterbox was exhausting.

After many medical tests, specialists, and time in hospital, the neurologist thought I may have Multiple Sclerosis (MS). Of course, this sent me into a state of anxiety. How was I going to cope with my family? I was too young, and I wanted to be there for my boys growing up. Then the medical diagnosis was made, and MS was ruled out. I was diagnosed instead with chronic fatigue syndrome, which was a new illness back then, and one that few knew much about. Being a new illness, there was no medical help for it other than anti-depressants. Against my better judgment, I took them for two weeks, but they made me worse than ever. I went off them against my doctor's advice as I couldn't function at all, and I cried on and off all day.

A mum from our local school who was an acquaintance arrived on our doorstep one day, and just handed me a book to read called *Take Responsibility for Your Own Health as Nobody Else Will*. These were the greatest words of advice I had ever received. I refer to her as a health angel since she had been through similar health issues and become well again. I sat on the couch by the fire wrapped up in a doona (my body was unable to maintain a warm temperature at the time) and read the book from cover to cover. It was about rebuilding your health from the cellular level, the building blocks – rehashing your diet, starting from the basics of food, slowly building the immune system to be strong again, lowering stress levels, and dealing with the emotions attached to illness.

Light bulb moment – reading this bought back many childhood memories of my father teaching us about the body and eating well for your health. Dad was a bit of a hippy and pretty much a vego at one stage in his life. He would say to us, "The body is able to heal itself if kept healthy and given the right food and supplements. The most amazing machine ever created and capable of healing itself!" He was a good singer, great bike rider and won many road races, and he loved the great Percy Cerutty's training and food programs, and the mind-power authors, Norman Vincent Peale. He also loved driving as a career – car carriers, buses and earthmoving machines as well.

Sadly, our dad was killed in a workplace accident at 42 years of age, so I never saw the benefits of what he put into place with his own health and how that would have played out as he matured. However, I rarely remember him visiting the doctor. He did suffer with migraines, and I think this was his motivation to find a cure through his interest in the benefits of whole foods and a healthy lifestyle.

I believe my father sent this lovely lady to deliver the book and the message as a reminder that my body could heal itself!

The medical profession had no answers, but suddenly, I found the motivation to do this myself. I was determined to get my body healthy again so I could be the best mum I could be to my boys – to care, love, play, read to, and watch them grow up!

I cleaned out my pantry and fridge of anything heavily processed as well as household cleaning chemicals. Everyone thought I had gone mad and had a nervous breakdown, but I knew I hadn't. I visited the local health food shop where my dad used to buy his healthy foods and discovered the same family was still running it. The owner commented that I must be revamping my diet for better health and asked if he could help. I answered a bit angrily, "Nobody can help me. I have to help myself." He handed me a card for a local homeopath practitioner who used a machine called Mora Therapy.

I thought it was strange since he didn't even know what was wrong with me. I think my dad had stepped in again, as this had been his and my grandparents' health food shop!

I made an appointment with the homeopath/mora therapist. The Mora machine gives a reading of the imbalances in the organs of the body. This was based on Chinese medicine and acupressure points of the fingers and toes. Diet changes were advised where needed – yeast and sugar-free plus managing lifestyle/

stress levels. This was supported by homeopathic drops; back then I was a guinea pig to trial large doses of garlic oil in capsules to kill off the massive yeast overgrowth (candida) in my body. Garlic oil scared off the friends for a short time but a small price to pay to have my life back!

It was the most amazing turning point in my life and my health. I never looked back! I had already stripped my diet and I made as many foods as I could, including nut butter, which was a feat back then. Food processors weren't what they are now, and yeast-free bread was like a brick! The homeopath and I made a great team, with her amazing health knowledge and healing work combined with the changes in my diet and dealing with the emotional and stress levels in my life, were all part of why my body was so sick. Combined, it all worked for me!

The neurologist who was treating me at the time was not keen on me trying alternative therapy. However, he also said that he had nothing else to offer medically, so the deal was I would try this and he would monitor me monthly.

It worked! After seven months, I woke one morning and felt like I had been tapped on the head by an angel, and I heard the words, "It's time to wake up now", and I did – back into life again. Within a very short time, I was driving the car again. My life and health were normal once more. And the only thing I had to monitor was spreading myself too thin, keeping my stress levels low, and eating healthy and as yeast-free as possible.

The neurologist was amazed at my progress after one month and commented that he couldn't wrap his Western head around this but it was working for me, so stick with it! He was happy to see me regaining my health. That's when it hit me. Wouldn't it be great if the Western and Eastern could meet halfway and work together for the health of all – balance between the two!

This is what I have done since – combining more Eastern than Western has worked for me!

However, I always have my yearly medical checks, such as iron, cholesterol, liver and kidney function, blood pressure, and any other check-ups for women with my local GP, who likes to always comment that I have the most expensive urine samples (due to my supplement intake). But my comeback is, "How often do you see me in your clinic?"

"Touché", is always his response. It's nice that we respect each other and can have a laugh! I still have a quarterly treatment with my homeopath and Mora therapist, an amazing practitioner, woman, associate, and friend. These quarterly treatments keep my body, mind, and emotions on track. If going on holidays or heading into a stressful time, I will have an extra treatment to keep my nervous system and body balanced and combine this with kinesiology sessions. Chiropractic has also been excellent for my health and which I have monthly, along with the occasional physiotherapy and massage if required. All of this, combined with my own daily health and simple exercise regime, now enables me to have balance in my life. It's been amazing for me!

Thank you to our family, friends, neighbours, community, and all the health practitioners who supported and helped us through a very challenging time – I am forever grateful!

On reflection, I had hit rock bottom with my health. My life was completely out of balance and overcompensating from my childhood experiences. I failed to speak up and ask for help. Trying to create a stable, safe, happy home and family and to be the perfect wife, supporting my husband and our business; being a mother, cook, cleaner and gardener; volunteering for school fundraising; basketball, footy, tennis, cricket, golf and surfing for our household of boys and their friends. I am not a martyr, just highlighting all the everyday things and multi-tasking we do as parents. I loved every minute of it but all the busyness and stress took its toll on my health! I forgot to take care of me!

> *"Mothers are the heartbeat*
> *of the household."*
>
> ~Tina Arena

I am so grateful I eventually healed, grew, and found balance in my life to experience the joy that resulted in giving our boys a good education, stability and life skills. They are all happy, healthy, well-adjusted men who have good work ethics and great careers. They enjoy life and all it offers. I am so proud they are honest, trustworthy, well-mannered men who respect women, and show empathy for others, and the world around them. I am so proud they have all become wonderful fathers and live fairly balanced lives — yes life has thrown curve balls at them as well, but they bounce back because they are not afraid to grow and learn. Quicker than I did!

Yes, there is reward for effort, and the three beautiful boys I gave birth to have now given me the gift of gorgeous grandchildren, a truly wonderful time of life being a Nanna to such amazing little souls so full of love and happiness. I embrace my son's lovely partners and have such gratitude and love for my ever expanding family.

Finding my true sole purpose in life has been wonderful, as has learning, discovering, accepting, and loving who I really am. Working through and healing all my past experiences has finally brought me peace, happiness, understanding, and joy with life!

I'm a woman who eventually got the best out of me. Not perfect, but now being the best I can be!

REMEMBER TO MAKE U NO. 1.
TAKE RESPONSIBILITY FOR YOUR LIFE,
HEALTH AND STRESS LEVELS OR YOUR WORLD
WILL COME CRASHING DOWN AROUND U!

Enjoy Your Journey!

Yes, life can be tough. You may be dealt some challenging hands at times; however, we can all make the choice to improve and grow, to learn from our experiences to create a happier life for ourselves. This will reflect on those around us. I refer to this as the ripple effect – work on U first, and your changes will ripple out to others. Think about when you throw a pebble into the water and the ripples move away from you! Interesting stuff!

"You either get better or you get bitter. It's simple. You either take what has been dealt to you and allow it to make you a better person, or you allow it to tear you down. The choice does not belong to fate. It belongs to you."

~power of positivity

We often find ourselves at the crossroads of life. Choosing the right path is up to you! Don't blame others, situations, or circumstances – that would be playing the victim or not taking responsibility. Victims love jumping on board the Drama Bus so everyone can feel sorry for them. Yes, the Drama Bus is a favourite story of mine. You have a choice: you can jump aboard the Drama Bus or stand there and wave it goodbye!

Life is a smoother, happier ride when you take responsibility and make good, positive choices to improve your life. Avoid riding the Drama Bus or playing the Blame Game. Taking responsibility is growth.

You don't need to remain a victim of your circumstances, thoughts or emotions. You have a choice everday to change – the choice is yours; it is up to U!

Never regret mistakes along the way because they are our greatest lessons. Learn from them and move on. When you have a shot at something, whether it works or not, there are no regrets, just lessons. Don't keep repeating the same mistakes unless, of course, you really didn't learn the lesson the first time!

Never let age be a barrier to experiencing or achieving anything. Wisdom and experience are wonderful gifts as we mature. **Don't make others the centre of your world. Be the centre of your own world and radiate out to others. This will then have an amazing ripple effect.**

You can choose to invite others to share your world as you wish. Don't keep negative/toxic/draining people in your life as they will only bring you down. They choose not to grow and don't want you to either as that creates change and that's a big, scary word to those who can't let go!

Change your attitude, thoughts, and beliefs. Then watch your world, and things will start to change around you! Those changes may be subtle or big, but they all have impact.

Life is not perfect. We, as humans, are not perfect. Some may like to project that they are. However, we are all part of nature and nature is not perfect either. Look at the plants, trees, sky and clouds. Nothing is exactly the same or perfect. Everything changes with the seasons. And yet, we often look at nature and only see perfection. We need to learn to bend and flex in the wind.

It's seeing the beauty and balance in all areas of your life that is perfect!

This book did not come about overnight but after many, many years of my own experiences and putting what I learnt into action. Oh yes, I have slipped up many times along the way and still do sometimes but now it's quicker and easier to get back on my bike and work towards a healthier, happier, more balanced life for me!

My journey has given me the healing gifts to support you on finding who you are and discovering your own life balance.

I have personally made each and every one of these changes in my life over many years – my learning journey. However, I have created this journal so you can achieve and make changes in your life in an easier, more streamlined way to achieve life-long results. I hope that sharing what I have learnt (and continue to learn) will help you to make the right choice for YOU.

TO BE THE BEST U!

"My goal is not to be better than anyone else, but to be better than I used to be."

~Wayne Dyer

CHAPTER 1

NOW CREATE YOUR OWN STORY...

"The best project you will ever work on is YOU, because you generate a ripple effect that impacts on everyone around you!"

~Dr Libby

NOTE TO ME:

Take Action: purchase a nice journal with blank pages for any notes or action for change in your life. Then have fun ticking them off as you achieve each one. Keep this journal so you can reflect on it later and celebrate how far you have come!

NOW write on the first page

This is My New Life Story of Choices and Changes for ME!

Be kind to yourself! Creating the best U isn't always easy, and making changes is challenging but so worth it!

"Happiness is the new rich. Inner peace is the new success. Health is the new wealth. Kindness is the new cool."

~Calm App

WARNING

Be kind to yourself during the process.

The guidance and changes for being the best U don't need to be made all at once. They are best done one step, one day, one week, one month at a time. Break it down and remove any pressure or stress you may put on yourself.

If you try to look too far ahead you may have trouble achieving your goals, and then what do we do? Give up before we see results. Sound familiar?

Make this light, fun, achievable, and enjoyable for U! Reward yourself when you reach each goal, then set a new one for the following week or month.

Important notes: you may not need to make all the changes I suggest. Just tweak a few areas to improve your flow and balance in life.

However, you may truly be ready and have the courage to step into the arena and make *all* the changes, but not all at once. Keep it simple – one step at a time.

You may notice I repeat some things in different subjects, and I do this purposefully. Repetition assists your subconscious into acceptance.

Learn from this read and take as little or as much as you need to improve your life. Even if you only make one or two changes, it's worth the effort!

Remember to work at your own pace with no pressure whatsoever. But for changes to really make an impact, you will have to **stop procrastinating, and take action for change to happen.**

Please don't beat yourself up if you drop the ball every now and then while making the changes, as some can be quite challenging. It's ok! Just get back on your bike the next day and start peddling towards a better U!

Remember, I'm no better or no less than U – I'm still learning and growing every day too!

I am very happy to share my vulnerabilities and experiences to assist and support you to grow and learn in a more streamlined way than I did. My passion and purpose is sharing the tools and strategies that have worked for me, my clients, and now U.

Take what works for you and your lifestyle. Have clear, easy and obtainable goals – or results I like to call them – and work towards them one step at a time.

However, once you start to make some changes, there will be a flow-on effect in other areas of your life. The ripple or flow-on effect will encourage and motivate you to keep going. I'm not saying I am going to be completely protected from ill health or my body letting me down in years to come, but I know that at least I've given it my best shot to live a healthy, happy life in body, mind, and spirit while I have the opportunity.

One precious life.
Make the most of it!

"No matter how many mistakes you make or how slow your progress is, you are still way ahead of everyone who isn't trying."

~author unknown

Dear Me,

I often compare my body and life to what's on TV, social media, magazines and those around me. But today, I am going to commit to having the strength and courage to be my best me - not anyone else's version of me. I will make me a priority. I will focus on self-love, self-worth, self-compassion and celebrate all of me and who I am - yes, all my toned and squishy bits - because I am important, and I now totally love and respect me.

I love me for the unique person I am!

♡

I ....

now commit to being the Best Me!

....

SIGNATURE

*Clarity comes from
Action not thought –
enjoy working through
the action pages.*

OK NOW,
LET'S GET
STARTED!

CHAPTER 2

THRIVE & SHINE

Thrive and Shine Health is my natural health studio. This is where my passion for Kinesiology, Qest4 Bioresonance and PSYCH-K is – supporting and guiding others to feel healthier and happier. Learning more about their health, growing, moving forward less stressed and anxious, feeling more confident, loving the unique person they are for a more balanced, positive life!

Isn't Thrive and Shine how we all want to feel!

Thriving is to become resilient, flourish, grow, prosper

"You may have missed the boat to a better life in the past, but never allow the past to keep you down and out. If you want to thrive, this is the time."

~Goodreads

Shining is to feel radiant, bright, full of positive energy, happy

"Stars do not pull each other down to be more visible; they shine brighter."

~Goodreads

ACTION

HOW DO U SEE YOURSELF?

Go on, look in the mirror and really be honest. What do you see? Bet you only see the not-so-perfect bits!

Ok, now write down how you see yourself: body, mind, personality – then ask your partner or close friend to write down how they see U! Swap lists and take note.

I'm guessing what they see won't be what U saw in the mirror. Now, that is all about to change!

Keep both lists in the back of this book or your journal and you will be checking in again at the end of this read.

Yes, by the end of this book, if you follow my guidance and invest some time on your health, happiness and discovering U, your search for a more balanced life will happen. The original list and image of how you saw yourself in the mirror will change. In fact, you may not even remember the old U!

From my years of experience, beauty is about making the best of your best and not–so-best bits, including fitness levels and healthy eating that suit you and your lifestyle; hair and make-up (even if it's just a little mascara and lipstick daily). Or you may look fabulous and happy with some sun block and little lip gloss or none at all. Your choice for U.

When it comes to your style, we don't have to be a slave to fashion. It can be exhausting and expensive. Choose what suits you best with your lifestyle, body shape, and then clear out the wardrobe. Hold garments up to you and ask: 'Does this lift my energy? Or, do I feel low energy?' Yes, you got it! Remove all the low energy and of course those things that don't fit anymore. Set up a basic, easy, mix-and-match selection of clothes for home, work and your social life, and maybe an outfit U feel very special in. For each season, add a little piece or two from the season's on-trend colours to give your wardrobe a boost. There are so many inexpensive options available to us now, so have fun with it and feel good!

Rule: if you buy one or several garments or pairs of shoes, remove the same amount from your old wardrobe to keep U and your wardrobe feeling beautifully balanced! Peel back a bit, keep everything simple and easy. Embrace the joy of slowing down a little.

Develop a food plan that supports your body and health. Feel comfortable and happy with who U are at any age by laughing and seeing the positive and funny side of life!

Learn to laugh at yourself!

Stop the sabotage. Start being kind to yourself, which means you need to put a little time into loving, caring, and accepting U!

That's what real beauty is: 'beauty from within and loving the one you're with – U!'

"I can't think of any better representation of beauty than a woman who is unafraid to be herself."

~Emma Stone

WISE WORDS IN THE WORLD OF TODAY!

Let's teach our daughters it's not about being beautiful.

Teach them to be bold, silly, strong, confident, independent, intelligent, brave, and fierce.
Be real in a world full of fake.

Let's Redefine Beauty.

~Whole Self Help

"Beauty begins the moment you decide to be yourself."

~Coco Chanel

CHAPTER 3

WHAT IS BALANCE?

'An even distribution of something that allows it to remain upright, steady, and stable where different things are equal or in the correct proportions.'

So now is your opportunity to discover where your life is out of balance!

Seriously, you wouldn't have picked up this book if it wasn't!

Invest some time and sort it out. Where are U out of balance? And if you can't see the forest for the trees, then ask someone close to you – a friend or partner, to be really honest and help you see where. Write your own list or maybe ask them to join you and write a list for each other to assist both of you to balance out your lives!

Striking Balance

Balance is not something you aim to achieve and that's it. It is a balancing act, adjusting often – even daily – to try and bring life back to balance. It's a real juggle, but if you are aware of it and motivated to find balance as often as possible, regularly making a point of correcting things when they become out of balance, then the quicker it will become routine in your daily life.

Self-regulation is connected to your resilience. Balance your time, energy, and ambitions. Awareness is the key; stop, pull things back, take action, and your life will flow better.

How many times do people become sick or even terminally ill before they realise how much their life and stress levels were out of balance? We hear stories of how they have adjusted their lives, lived more simply, enjoyed more of the gifts around them, and often found balance and peace that they may never have felt in years or ever. So why wait till you're sick or stressed to the max? Start now!

This will be different for everyone. So work towards finding your own personal balance!

The Dalai Lama, when asked what surprised him most about humanity, he answered, '*Man, because he sacrifices his health in order to make money. Then he sacrifices money to recuperate his health. And then he is so anxious about the future that he does not enjoy the present. The result being that he does not live in the present or the future. He lives as if he is never going to die, and then dies having never really lived.*'

ACTION

WHERE IS MY LIFE OUT OF BALANCE?

- ☐ Health . . . .
- ☐ Weight . . . .
- ☐ Exercise . . . .
- ☐ Attitude . . . .
- ☐ Time for me . . . .
- ☐ Personal/relationships . . . .
- ☐ Family/home . . . .
- ☐ Work . . . .
- ☐ Finances . . . .
- ☐ Fun/social/friendships . . . .

Who lifts my energy and is easy to be around? . . . .

. . . .

Who zaps my energy? . . . .

The idea is to grow the people, places, and activities that lift your energy and make you feel good. Just because some people may be family or friends, if they choose not to treat you with love, respect and support, it shows their lack of love and respect for themselves. The tip is to reduce time with them or if very toxic, delete them from your life so they can learn and deal with their own stuff.

Delete or change the energy zappers that leave you feeling low, tired, drained, or stressed. Write or highlight the energy lifters, and put a line through the zappers – move them on!

Being aware is the beginning! Now, place a note somewhere you can read daily just the word: '**Balance**'. It can be next to your toothbrush, the dash of your car, your desk at work, or on your phone. Put reminders everywhere so you start naturally adjusting to bring life into balance.

Once you are aware and you put this into regular practise, it becomes part of your daily life. Our lives are forever moving and changing with many outside influences. That's why balance can never be fully achieved 100%. It is always a work in progress. Some days it really works, while other days it becomes more challenging. Days or weeks that give you that feeling 'how am I going to get through all this?' – **Stop**, and re-evaluate. What can I say **NO** to? What can I drop off my plate so I can achieve the most important things and breathe? You, your life, and those around you will benefit from this, so share with others close to you to join in the fun of finding balance! Ok, you're now **aware** – yeah!

Time to gain **insight!** You have listed the reasons where you don't have balance. Now, your choice to write on the previous Action page or into your own journal *why*, and don't blame others or circumstances.

Accept **change**. Choose from your list above, highlight the area that is most out of balance, and write down one **action** next to it that you can change. Then work your way through the other areas. Of course, you may only have one area, or you can choose to work on multiple areas – it doesn't matter. But it may help to commit to this change by sharing your action with someone close if you wish to keep *you* accountable. Be **grateful**. Just sit for a few moments each day and focus on what you *have*, not what you *don't have*. This will bring balance to the mind.

Start a **plan**. Book a little relaxation or 'me' time each day. It could be as simple as a walk in nature, closing your eyes for a few minutes, sitting quietly and focusing on your breathing, having a nice cuppa/lunch break away from technology and your desk with no interruptions, or dancing to your favourite music. The point is to let go, and do it daily.

Be **present and turn off**. Have one activity a day in which you are totally present. Disconnect from everything else and focus on just this one thing, be it brushing your teeth, cooking, exercising, walking or communicating with someone one-on-one are some examples. Being present means just focusing totally on that one thing while you're doing it.

Loosen up and laugh! Laugh at yourself, have fun, don't take life too seriously, and loosen up. We are all here for a good time.

Your body. Eat healthy, exercise, meditate, and – here is the big one – sleep well and for long enough. Shut down all devices two hours before bed. Remember that when the body is balanced, so is the mind.

Focus on U! Learn to say **no**. It's ok. Don't just say yes to things out of obligation or for being a people pleaser. Saying no gets easier once you start, and you will feel so relieved.

"A balanced life is one in which you're living from your deepest values in a way that is self-renewing, stimulating, and satisfying."

~Phillip Moffit

ENJOY FINDING YOUR OWN STYLE OF BALANCE SO U CAN THRIVE AND SHINE!

"And I said to my body softly,
'I want to be your friend!'
It took a long breath and replied,
'I have been waiting my whole life for this.'"

~Nagyirah Waheed

CHAPTER 4

BODY IMAGE -LOVING U

The first and most important area we must deal with is LOVING U!

It all begins with loving ourselves. We all need to feel loved, be loved, and give love. This will be your greatest challenge but the most rewarding, and this will be the start of the changes. Once we learn to begin to love ourselves, the rest will be easier. This is where you will experience the most profound changes. I know, it took me years before I discovered this and once I put this into daily practise, so many other areas in my life became easier. My attitude and awareness towards many things also improved dramatically.

"Don't forget to love her. The little girl you used to be. Perhaps she lies within you – untucked, sleeping peacefully."

~Kiana Llanos

WARNING

Those close to you will either notice the changes and be delighted and supportive. Or, they will be negative and want to pull you back to where you were because it highlights the changes they are resisting. Some see it as: 'how dare you love yourself? It's selfish and self-centred'. I think of it this way: if you come crashing down with your health, your family and your world will also come crashing down around you. So doesn't it make sense to love and care for yourself first? Then you can support others. Think about it. It makes a lot of simple sense, and boy I wish I'd learnt this in my early-twenties! Call it selfless and the greatest gift you can give yourself!

Be brave, be strong, and step forward! Embrace loving U and your life will change!

Unfortunately, our upbringing, society, and the media have the effect of making us feel unworthy. We need to be everything to everybody. We deal with work, family, partners, etc. We are not no. 1, and that should be reversed. We must be no. 1 with our health, fitness, and regular me time, so we are at the top of our game to support others. It's just not good enough. This is so sad because self-worth should not be determined by others and we should feel that it's ok to love and feel good about ourselves. I don't mean this in an egotistical, show-off kind of way; just feeling good about U inside and out!

So embrace and love all the bits of your body - squashy or toned - love them equally. Eat and exercise because you love U and not because you don't like U!

Give your body what it deserves: the time to exercise or relax; eat healthy, nutritious foods balanced with some occasional indulgent treats. It's all about balance and feeling good. Life is to be enjoyed. A good, healthy meal with a nice glass of wine or dessert shared with friends or family brings joy!

Note: this is not permission to eat a whole cake or drink a bottle of wine. No guilt attached. Just feel happy and love this one important life. *Really, what have U got to lose? Feeling better is the reward!*

Just Show Up For U!

In our everyday life, we always start with good intentions. Sometimes, life diverts us from our path and that's ok! If you sleep through the alarm one morning, skip that early exercise, or eat unhealthy for a day, just get back on your bike and start again the next morning! As long as you show up for U each day and keep trying, the 'doing' part will become easier and more natural. Be kind to yourself and keep trying just for U!

"Life is like riding a bike, to keep your balance you must keep moving forward."

~Albert Einstein

ACTION

Look at your body naked in the mirror. Oooh, now that's a bit scary! If it's too challenging to look at your whole body first up, then each day expose one body part at a time until you can look at your whole body. It should only take about a week. Consider this: you look at your face every day and it's part of your body. So be brave and really look at your body even if it's just a few seconds – front and back. Now, each day after you shower, dry off, look in the mirror, smile and say:

"I love my body. I love me!"

~Louise Hay

Don't get stuck on the squishy bits because we all have them. Just love your body as a whole. This isn't easy and there may be tears at first, but it feels so good once you achieve it and make it your daily routine. I still do this, and it really does change your whole mindset about yourself, your body image, feeling comfortable with who you are and how you see life. Truly loving yourself is the key; it creates a ripple effect in all areas of your life. So start now!

Note: Don't think too much and just write down:

Which parts of my body do I love? . . . .

. . . .

Which parts need more love and acceptance? . . . .

. . . .

Love Your Body.
It's Time to Commit to U!

After you have achieved this exercise, you will start to wake up happier every day, look at your body, and say to yourself in the mirror: **I love me!**

Feel grateful for all the amazing things our body does for us every day: like our heart beating and our lungs breathing, our body is an awesome machine! Without even thinking, our body does all of this. Be thankful!

Warning: As soon as we come under stress and become negative, we become harsh on ourselves and our body image. That little voice in your head starts chatting negatively. **The more U judge the less U love!** Learn to nurture your body just like a garden. Care for it, feed it, and give it your full focus and attention. What does the garden do when you give it lots of the right food, water, love, and care? THRIVES!

GO ON, START THRIVING, NOT JUST SURVIVING!

CHAPTER 5

SELF-SABOTAGE
AND SELF-WORTH

'Sabotage: Deliberately destroying, damaging, or obstructing something.'

Sound familiar? That little, critical voice in your head saying, 'You can't do this and achieve that. You're not good enough, not smart enough, not educated enough. What do you think you are trying to achieve beyond your limitations?' Oh, that critical inner voice! How it destroys our self-worth and self-confidence! We can be our own worst enemy with all this negative self-talk, and it has the ability to rear its ugly head to stop us from moving forward in life and achieving our goals, dreams, and happiness.

Self-sabotage destroys our self-worth!

I'll let you in on a secret. We all have a habit of self-sabotage when we are challenged and trying to move forward. I have self-sabotaged so many times during my life because I didn't believe in myself. This all stemmed from my childhood. It's where we develop genetic patterns, but I'm here to share with you that they can be broken.

I had major self-sabotage tendencies while writing this book. In fact, it was the last subject I wrote as it was the most challenging for me, and I put up all the road-blocks of self-sabotage. A big one was avoidance. As this book was never ever on my life's agenda, I didn't believe in me, in my ability to write it.

I creatively developed and wrote in my own style, drawing from the work with my clients and realising that I was able to successfully help them as I had experienced all the issues they presented. I have great empathy and found my passion – guiding others to let go, put the past behind them, and enjoy a better life being happy with who they are. I had travelled their paths with a positive result in discovering who I am, and I now enjoy a happier, healthier life.

It's taken me a lifetime to achieve this and I still have a lot of life yet to live. It's always a work in progress for me. I came to realise that if we are willing, we never stop learning and growing. This was not achieved on my own. I was treated by and I listened to health practitioners. I studied, learnt, took action, and I grew into me!

As I wrote on this subject that is close to my heart, my tears flowed until I finished writing, I had to constantly work on myself to get through this tough subject, and I did it!

See, I am only human, too. I struggle and stumble occasionally. However, the difference now is that I recognise it and work on it immediately no matter how difficult I find it to be. I adjust quicker, break through those road-blocks more easily, and sometimes they turn out to be just a speed bump. Once I got through this, I wiped the tears and the awareness made me laugh. I felt so much better believing in me, my work, and in writing this book for U!

As a Kinesiologist, it is one of the most common things I assist clients with. I know it so well myself. I understand and have the experience, empathy, and wisdom to guide them to a more positive belief in themselves, who they are, and what they truly can achieve.

We often don't even realise we are self-sabotaging. We just believe we are inadequate, fill our heads with more negative messages, and believe our lack of success in any area of our life is a complete lack of our own adequacies. It's not. It's our belief system. Believe in U no matter what your past or present have been dictating. U have the ability within to change! Your self-worth is non-negotiable. U deserve complete respect.

"You can't hate yourself happy. You can't criticize yourself thin. You can't shame yourself wealthy. Real change begins with self-care and self-love."

~Jessica Ortner

Signs You Are Sabotaging

You are self-sabotaging when things come to a halt. You feel you have the ability, energy, and desire, but there is no rational reason stopping you from moving forward – it's usually just U!

Procrastination: you keep putting something off, you start but never quite finish, you feel unmotivated, and you do many other tasks to avoid the one you should be focusing on.

Worry: you constantly worry over small things that really shouldn't matter. There is the fear of failure – you worry what others will think, doubt your abilities, and stress over trying to achieve something for U.

Destruction: you destroy or display aggressive communication with family, friends, or work colleagues that can play out as anger, resentment, and even jealousy due to your own feelings of inadequacy.

Low self-worth: you allow others to put you down, take to heart unfair criticism, and exaggerate other people's achievements, which you think diminishes your own.

We make decisions from fear or love. Most of us come from fear, which is often disguised as being practical. What appears to be so far out of our reach or impossible to achieve is only because we don't believe in ourselves or out of fear of asking for it!

*"Everything you want is on the
other side of fear."*

~Jack Canfield

Recognise your self-sabotage pattern. It may be one or a blend of several factors. However, you must overcome the negative self-talk to build your self-confidence and self-worth.

Building self-love and self-worth within gives good grounding for creating strong boundaries. Create self-compassion, stop judging and putting yourself down; instead, put your hand on your heart and give yourself the love, compassion and kind words you would give to a friend. Be your own best friend!

*"It is our light, not our darkness,
we are frightened of."*

~ Nelson Mandela

ACTION

RECOGNISING YOUR CYCLE
OF SELF-SABOTAGE

"The temptation to quit is greatest just before you are about to succeed."

~Chinese proverb

What is my self-sabotage pattern? (avoid, delay, procrastinate, anger)

. . . .

What does my inner-critic say to me?

. . . .

What has fear stopped me from achieving? (personally, health, career, family, friends)

. . . .

Where do I lack motivation?

. . . .

What goals or results would you like to achieve but have never been able? (keep it simple)

. . . .

Why are you procrastinating, avoiding making a decision, and blaming others? (what is your fear)

. . . .

NOW LET YOUR LIGHT SHINE!

Break the Self-Sabotage Cycle

Well done! U have recognised your 'how' and 'where' of self-sabotage.

When the negative self-talk starts, write down notes to yourself, even the silly thoughts. Try and identify by imagining or recalling what you were thinking last time that negative inner voice started. Is it from childhood, school, a parent, friend or partner? Helping to identify the origin brings awareness.

Challenge your thinking. What you have discovered sets the inner voice chatting negatively at U. Were there previous unsuccessful attempts that are preventing you from moving forward? Fear of failure often ignites negativity.

Tip: press the delete button in your mind every time a negative thought or comment enters then replace with a positive.

Now you have identified the cause,
U can freely move forward!

What can I say to me that is positive and supportive? It may be just a word. Say an affirmation, write it down, and put it somewhere, or many places, where you can read it regularly – toothbrush, undies drawer, car dashboard, or inside your work desk. What is my positive support word or sentence? What would I say to a best friend?

Look at others who seem to achieve great results. They

usually have great belief in themselves, and that's what U need to create in U – self-belief! Not easy but give it a go!

Ask for support if you need it from those close to you and those who truly believe in U and your goals. Accept their support and positive feedback, or seek out a practitioner who can assist with support to clear the negative chatter and give you tools to assist you with staying on a positive pathway of believing in U.

It's not easy turning self-sabotage around. I still sometimes struggle with it. However, I now recognise it and call on the tools I need to change it. Believe in yourself and your abilities no matter what anyone else thinks.

Stay in your own lane!

Self-sabotage is an easy pattern to fall into. After many years, it becomes a comfort zone, so we don't have to deal with the scary stuff.

It's a difficult habit to break but once you are aware and you develop your strategies to kick it in the butt, your self-esteem, self-worth, and confidence will shine through for a more satisfying, fulfilling, and happier life.

We need to grow a more compassionate, loving, grounded way toward ourselves and start to choose and recognise what you really want for U and not what others want. Choose your own destiny! U don't need validation or approval from others – just U!

Align yourself daily with positive beliefs in yourself and what you would like to achieve. Flip the negative inner voice to a positive inner voice – Yes I Can or Yes I Am!

Be prepared. You may falter along the way as this is one of the hardest habits to break. Stop beating yourself up and just let go!

Get back on your bike and start pedalling forward in the right direction the next day.

"Our deepest fear is not that we are inadequate. Our deepest fear is that we are powerful beyond measure. It is our light, not our darkness, that most frightens us. We ask ourselves – who am I to be brilliant, talented, gorgeous? Who are you not to be – you are a child of God!"

~ Nelson Mandela

REMEMBER

"You are a glorious, abundant, majestic soul ready to live your greatest life."

~author unknown

CHAPTER 6

PERFECTION

I am so over the media presentation of perfection and the so-called perfect way our lives should be – from perfect face, skin, hair, body, fashion, families, homes... the list goes on. It's a hard gig. Like carrying a suit of armour. It takes a lot of energy trying to be perfect! But I'll let you in on something: there is no perfect in anything!

We often compare our bodies and lives to what we read in magazines or view on TV, movies, and those around us. Remember, these are mostly photoshopped and airbrushed with a team of experts preparing the models or actors for their shoots, plus it takes hours and hours of creating the so-called perfection.

Our bodies and lives are not perfect. Nature is not perfect and we are part of nature. Are all the plants and trees perfect? No. They grow uneven but balanced in an imperfect way. Sunrises, sunsets, and the clouds are not always the same. However, we look at the wonder of nature and see it as just perfect!

It's great we now have the 'odd bunch' of fruit and veggies appearing on the supermarket shelves, fruit markets, or in your own veggie garden. The way things naturally grow shows us that there is no perfection in nature, but it tastes just perfect. We are also part of nature, so why are we striving so hard and putting so much stress and pressure on ourselves to reach perfection?

Can you see the difference between perfection and just perfect?

Constant perfectionism creates constant low-level stress over time, and sometimes, a lifetime has the ability to create dis-ease in our bodies and minds. In the pursuit of perfection, STOP and think about what this is doing to your health, both mentally and physically. My personal view is that perfectionism is partnered with control, and the more we feel an area of our life is out of our control, whether it be physically or emotionally, the more we aim for more control. But control is mostly about fear!

Procrastination: you don't know where to start.

Perfectionism: you don't know when to ease your foot off the perfection peddle and stop!

Don't be confused with being a good organiser and being a perfectionist. Some of us are born to be organisers and good organisers can easily fall into the perfectionism role by over-organising.

Learn to let some things go and let others have some of the organisational control. Now, whether that meets your highest standards is not to be judged. Learn to handle it in a more diplomatic, delicate way. That doesn't mean redoing what others have done because that just demoralises people, and you won't get the best out of them. Moreover, that will not help take the stress and load off you if you redo or take back the allocated job. Praise them and guide them in how that could be improved next time if you need to, or let go and accept it without judgement.

We all make mistakes. That is where our greatest learning lies. Draw on your strengths and build on your lesser strengths from those around you. You actually disempower people by not allowing them some control, so allow them their power and ideas, and show their strengths so you both learn and grow.

"You don't inspire others by being perfect. You inspire them by how you deal with your imperfections."

~author unknown

So stop beating yourself up by striving for 'Perfection' and start working on 'Letting Go' – it's ok!

We have a habit, as humans, of seeing all our imperfections and forgetting to focus on all our positive traits. Embrace the beauty and the good in the beautiful, unique person that you are, and truly accept and feel comfortable with U. Try to put this into practise with those around you, challenge yourself to focus on their strengths. **The more we judge the less we love!**

Of course, this doesn't give you a ticket to be irresponsible with your health, exercise, or attitude.

Example: I have short legs and there's nothing I can do about it. But I learnt to love and be grateful for them and try to keep them strong because they are important to keep me upright and moving through my daily life.

It is the greatest gift in life you can give yourself. The sooner you accept and love U for who U are and stop aiming for perfection, the happier and more at peace U will become!

Why am I trying to strive for perfection? Give yourself permission to take your foot off the pedal and release the stress that comes with perfection. After all, what are we trying to prove to ourselves? Sometimes, this striving for perfection arises from feeling insecure about ourselves or feeling out of control, which again is fear-based.

Go on, take a good look at U and turn your so-called imperfections and negative attitude into positives by having gratitude and acceptance every day for your beautiful body, mind, health, spirit, and life.

Are we feeling insecure or inadequate or afraid of judgement? Is it recognition we are chasing or is it simply that we need to love who and what we are – warts and all – just like the 'odd bunch of veggies'?

We are all perfectly imperfect and that's Ok.

ACTION

Now take a long, slow, deep breath from your belly. Hold, slowly release, accept, and embrace. Repeat this a few times.

Be really honest and write a list of where you over-strive and put pressure on yourself or others for control or perfection.

- [ ] My body . . . .

- [ ] Exercise . . . .

- [ ] Relationships . . . .

- [ ] Career . . . .

- [ ] Family . . . .

- [ ] Friends . . . .

- [ ] Home . . . .

- [ ] Garden . . . .

- [ ] Friendships . . . .

- [ ] Entertaining . . . .

- [ ] Fashion . . . .

Why do I feel the need for perfection?

(fear, control, being judged, insecure)

. . . .

. . . .

. . . .

Under each area, make a note of how you can take your foot off the perfection pedal and work towards being better – not perfect – and begin to feel the flow of life!

*Life is more enjoyable
when you learn
to just Let Go!*

GO ON. BE BRAVE.
THE WORLD WON'T END.

CHAPTER 7

CHANGE

*"If you change the way you look at things,
the things you look at change."*

~Wayne Dyer

One guarantee in life is **change!** Yes, none of us like the thought of change and some adjust more easily to change than others. But you have two choices when it comes to this: **fight** it because you **fear** it and it feels so uncomfortable usually because you are not in control.

OR

Embrace it. Feel the fear and just go with it! Try to stop controlling and manipulating to make things work. Go with and trust the timing and flow of life. Believe and enjoy the process of change, you may be pleasantly surprised with what it may bring into your life!

Stop swimming against the tide. Go with it and experience how much easier life flows.

There is no blame here, but my childhood was what it was. However, it was my greatest lesson to be part of a poor, dysfunctional family, and I made a choice to change that for myself and my own family.

Health practitioners, GPs, and psychologists who have supported me during tough times over the years have all described me as an extremely resilient woman. I had never really thought of myself that way. However, while writing this book, I have realised that, yes, I am resilient. These are my lessons from childhood and my adult life when I got knocked down – and there have been so many of those times; I pick myself up, dust off, accept the changes, and move forward.

Example: you know when someone keeps attracting the same people into their lives or the same situations, 'Oh it always happens to me' or 'my life is stressful, crappy, and nothing ever changes'?

Some people will choose not to recognise or get the lessons, so be grateful when you do. Then, you don't need to repeat the same lesson over and again in different forms until you get it. Lightbulb moments I call them. Learning the lesson creates change for the better!

Yes, I am still learning lessons all the time. However, with wisdom and maturity, I recognise them a lot quicker, learn, and move forward easier. With any negative situation that now presents in my life, instead of saying, 'why is this happening to me?' I look at it and ask: 'what is my lesson in this situation?' It's been sent for a reason. It may be that I need to stand up for myself, speak up for myself, be more open to a person's view, listen more, be more patient, just let go, open my heart, or create stronger boundaries.

Of course, the other person has something to learn as well and theirs may be a very different lesson, but focus on your lesson and try to recognise it for what it is – good, bad or ugly – and make the **change**. It can be quite challenging or very simple. Try it next time something presents itself and ask, 'What is my lesson?' and see if you can recognise, rectify, and create **change for the better**.

Learning my lessons has made me resilient and a better person, mother, partner, friend, and health practitioner so *thank you childhood for all my lessons and the choices I made to change and enjoy a happier life!*

"If you're not learning something in this life, you might as well be dead."

~my awesome and wise grandfather, Jack

I hope my experiences of change can have an impact on your life. Sometimes, the smallest, consistent changes can have the greatest impact!

Good always comes from adversity.

We can never see it at the time but when you look back, you know why it happened. I use this quote often with my family, friends, and clients when they are going through challenging times – everything is sent to us for a reason. If you can recognise the reason and learn from it, you will move forward and life will be better. Always look forward not back.

You can't change your past but
you do have a choice every day
to change your future!

Challenges make you grow when things are feeling uncomfortable. It's a sign we are growing. Keep the changes simple, don't set the uncomfortable zone too high or you will be overwhelmed.

I keep repeating this because it's so important: take one step at a time, one change at a time. Don't try and change your whole world at once or you will create a meltdown!

START BY DOING ONE PUSH UP.
START BY DRINKING ONE EXTRA CUP OF WATER.
START BY PAYING TOWARDS ONE DEBT.
START BY READING ONE PAGE.
START BY MAKING ONE SALE.
START BY DELETING ONE OLD CONTACT OR EMAIL.
START BY WALKING ONE LAP.
START BY ATTENDING ONE EVENT.
START BY WRITING ONE PARAGRAPH.
START BY LETTING GO OF CONTROLLING ONE THING.
START TODAY AND REPEAT TOMORROW.
THIS IS HOW TO MAKE POSITIVE CHANGE HAPPEN!

~power positivity

ACTION

Small changes help you move towards a greater life that flows more easily.

What is draining your energy and motivation in life?

Really think: what is blocking it? Is it me? Am I sabotaging myself by not allowing time for me? Or, is it because I don't feel I am worthy or deserve to have a better life? I feel life has to be hard, so does it mean I've become hard on myself?

. . . .

. . . .

. . . .

. . . .

Where and how would I like to make change happen for me?

. . . .

. . . .

What issues have I been struggling with?

. . . .

. . . .

What are my lessons in these situations?

....

....

What changes do I need to make to be positive and move forward?

....

....

Do I just need to let go of the resistance, surrender, and trust the process?

....

....

"Growth may be painful, change may be painful, but being stuck where you are not happy is even more painful."

~Anonymous

CHAPTER 8

CHOICES

"Your life will work better when you take full responsibility for your choices."

~Anonymous

Just think for a moment how many choices we make during our day!

Food: do I want to eat to feel energised, healthy, well, and reduce some kilos? **OR** do I want to feel crappy after over-indulging eating stodgy, sweet, fatty foods, too many cigarettes, or alcohol?

Exercise: do I take a walk, go to the gym, stretch and move my body, or meditate so I feel energised and clear-headed to start the day? **OR** do I just roll over and hit the snooze button then drag myself through the day?

Allow yourself one day a week 'alarm free'.

The choice is yours on how you would like to feel.

Family: no matter how our families are made up, be it the family you were born into or a blended family, they are always an interesting mix of personalities. As far as I'm concerned, all families experience dysfunction at times, some just more than others, but that's a whole subject on its own.

Our choices are how we react, respond, respect, and deal with family members. Issues that may arise are tricky ones, but you have a choice to **react** or **respond!**

React: initial knee-jerk reaction **OR** take a breath, wait a moment, think, then respond.

Respond in the most positive, non-reactive way for the good of all. Of course, this doesn't excuse some people's behaviour, and you can't change them. However, your choice and attitude can change for you. As I say, this is a really tough one at times, but you still have a choice.

Personal relationships: love, respect, compatibility, communication, honesty, trust, family and commitment – are you on the same page with these values in life? Have you got each other's back? Can you freely express yourself? Is there equal decision-making, especially with finances? Is there a compromised balance with your incomes? Is one being too controlling of the other?

The answer to these questions can be deal breakers in most relationships. We have a choice to work on improving these qualities if you want your relationship to last. **OR**, if the relationship is really lacking these qualities, there is no hope and you will be really unhappy – get out! Remove draining, toxic people or issues from your life; they only drag you down.

Work: this is your chosen career, hours of work, those you work with, or manage as a team. Maybe you work on your own, but this is still a choice. You can choose to work to your best but not perfection; there is a difference. Remember to inspire those around you. **OR**, sit day after day feeling unsatisfied, unfulfilled, unhappy, complaining and feeling stuck. But you always have a choice to change your situation. Apply for other positions, retrain part-time in a new career path, or develop extra skills you may need to move forward in your current career while still working.

Find your purpose and thrive doing what U love! When you love the work you do, the money will follow.

Finances: this can be a minefield for some of us, and we can all stick our heads in the sand at times about money. However, we have a choice to take control and manage our finances to support our lifestyle.

What are my choices? Ignore it, allow debt to pile up, and feel too stressed to even look at your bank statements. **OR**, seek advice and put strategies in place to reduce/eliminate debt. Your spending and lifestyle may need adjusting for a little while, but it will be worth it to take control of your finances and reduce the stress. Seeking help is not a failure. It's stepping up and making a choice!

Note: Scott Pape, known as the 'Barefoot Investor' in Australia, has great advice and books to read with simple, down-to-earth actions to put into place to assist with your finances. David Bach's *The Latte Factor*, is a quick and easy read to get you started, and he has also written many other books for different stages of our financial lives.

Holidays as regular recharge: have you become a slave to the grind, never taking that regular break to restore and recharge? You may think, 'no, too much to do, no time to take a break'. Well, yes you do! It just takes some forward thinking and planning. Really sit and look outside the square and ask others for help if you can't see the forest for the trees.

This doesn't mean you have to take an overseas trip each year. Try a road trip or a holiday at home and be a tourist in your own town/city – it's fun! If your career doesn't allow for longer breaks, take a long weekend once a month or plan every three months to take a week off – this has great recharge benefits. **OR**, you may have to plan around school holidays. I know that's busy but it can be fun joining in the kid's activities. Stay in your pyjamas, make pancakes, watch a fun movie, set up board games, or walk or ride together. It's still a break from work and daily routines.

You may need to approach your employer or your team and delegate more, negotiate better work hours, or job share with someone. If approached in a positive manner, there is usually a way. If you're self-employed, plot your time off in your diary/planner. Clients understand that we all need a break to recharge just like they do!

Again, you are making a choice to give yourself recovery and recharge time before your battery runs flat and have it negatively effect those around you – family, partners, and friends. As the old marketing quote goes, we must all have **'work, rest, and play'** to really enjoy our life and those we love to share it with.

The choice is yours to be grumpy and tired or have a break, lighten up, and have some fun!

Here's one of my strategies for choice making. Think about the choice you are trying to make. 'Is this in my highest good?' When you think about the issue and the choices, close your eyes and really tap into how it makes you feel emotionally.

Heavy, like trudging through mud, feeling knots, or having an upset stomach **OR**, **light** with anticipated excitement and joy!

If you feel heavy, it may not be for you, or the timing is wrong. But if you feel light, excited, and happy, it's right!

Note: Don't confuse heaviness and fear because we can just fear the unknown at times. Of course, if we are making a big major life/career decision, we need to write a list of pros and cons plus do all the background research and professional advice if needed, then try this process.

If we all relied more on this simple exercise known as our gut instinct or inner knowing, we would only be working towards our highest good. Of course, the choices we make also have the ripple effect on those around us. However, my experience is if you truly make the right choices for U –and feel light and excited but grounded – it can only have a positive effect on your world and those around you.

"If it is to be, it is up to me!"

~unknown

ACTION

Where would I like to make change happen and how?
Start small and you can grow bigger, and then you can
adjust to the change happening.

....

....

Where would I like to make some new choices and how?
(Refer to the above list and remember your choices:
respond or react)

....

....

....

CONGRATS,
YOU'RE NOW WELL
ON THE WAY!

CHAPTER 9

ATTITUDE IS EVERYTHING!

The rest of my life is the best of my life!

Drop the thoughts 'I will never get there' when thinking about whether you can save, exercise, lose weight, improve your life or current situation, or get work-life balance!

Flip it to 'How can I work towards achieving it or changing my situation?'

You can say 'Why?' and play the victim, or you can flip it to 'Why not?' and give it a positive shot!

Start small and build on it. The universe or life will not support you unless U step up to the plate and start taking action. Show yourself and the world that you are serious with making change. No one hands anything to you on a platter. If they did, there would be no challenge and you would never truly appreciate, be grateful for, or learn anything!

90% RULE PUTS YOU IN 100% CONTROL

*I have a choice every day of
what my attitude will be.*

I cannot change my past.

*I cannot change the
attitudes of others.*

I cannot change the inevitable.

*The only thing I can change
is my attitude!*

*"Life is 10% what happens to me
and 90% how I react."*

~Chuck Swindoll

Remember, try not to be overwhelmed. Once you look at the big picture, this can happen so easily.

I recommend you start gradually. You might want to start with your attitude towards life. **Do U say more negative or positive statements?** Consider when friends are going on holidays – what do you say? 'Isn't that great for them? Hope they have a safe and fun time'. **OR**, 'Wish it was me. I never get a break'.

Start by pushing the delete button in your mind on the negative statements and try to change each thought or statement into positive ones. Yes, we all wish we could go on that holiday, lose weight, feel fitter, or happier as well. However, instead of having a negative attitude and comparing ourselves to others, flip the thought to:

'Yes, I'd love a break, too. How can I work towards this, what attitude or changes can I make if I want to have a holiday, lose weight, exercise, or have more time for me?'

Remember to start simple. Reduce how many times you go to a café or buy a take-away coffee, lunch or takeaway dinners in a week, and put this money plus your small change in a lovely jar for holiday spending or a night out. Got the idea?

Now set yourself a 90-day challenge, the money you used to spend on these things put into your...

Fun Fund! Get everyone involved. You can have one big jar or personal jars.

Now, put your brain and attitude into action and start making positive change! One step at a time and you will get there.

ACTION

Make a to-do list on the action page for each area of your life that needs a change in attitude.

☐ Food Plan . . . .

☐ Exercise . . . .

☐ Stress Levels . . . .

. . . .

☐ Communication. . . . .

. . . .

☐ Relationships/Family/Friends. . . . .

. . . .

☐ Career . . . .

☐ Finances. . . . .

☐ Regular Recharge Breaks/Holiday. . . . .

. . . .

Focus on one thing at a time or you will become scattered and not achieve the desired results. Once you feel you have momentum and feel good with one change, then start on another area of your life. **Break it down step by step and keep it simple** or you will become overwhelmed and give up easily. I know I keep repeating this but it's important!

Maybe each month, depending on how you're feeling, introduce another change. Keep checking on your attitude towards life, situations, and other people.

How am I feeling now about this? Light Energy compared to 'How did I previously feel?' Heavy Energy.

Note the changes. Some take a little while to get that light feeling, depending on how long the negativity has been sitting there. Be really aware. It is very easy to go back to our comfort zone of how we used to feel or do things, as this is where it feels safe. But this is **sabotage.**

It truly is harder to make changes than stick with what we know – your choice!

The idea is to gradually move through each change one at a time, which will then really consolidate a complete lifestyle shift. You may be surprised once you start changing one area of your life, it may flow into other areas.

Be aware of the changes that may happen in your world. You may feel happier or notice that life is flowing better. Negative people or situations may decrease or when someone asks you, 'How are you?' your response may be 'I'm having a really good day' or 'I'm feeling great today' instead of 'I'm so busy, got so much on my plate, I'm so stressed, and all these things are wrong'.

Here's a lovely story I read a few years ago. A parent was explaining the difference of positive and negative to a child. *There were two wolves fighting, one was full of negative emotions – angry, mad; the other held positive emotions – happy, kind, loving. The child asked which wolf won? The wise reply was the one you fed the most!*

Negative responses attract negative energy.

Positive responses attract positive energy.

It's ok to NOT have every minute of every day full. Give yourself permission to take stock and really look at changing how you're living your life and how it is affecting U and those around you!

Taking positivity to the extreme is so not necessary.

Don't fall for the Pollyanna Syndrome where the person runs around, constantly smiling and saying how wonderful and busy everything is in their life. The truth is that they are totally exhausting, their idea is to project to the world and anyone who listens that everything is totally amazing in their life. But scratch the surface a little and it's often not the case.

You know the person who enters the room over-the-top happy and positive, isn't everything wonderful, my life is just amazing and often give you an air kiss then launch into 'all about them' stories. Their emotional mission is to suck the life out of a room and take everyone else's energy for themselves, which is a reflection of their own low self-worth, insecurities and great need to refill their self-esteem tank.

Of course, it's often all smoke and mirrors. You know they're not really sincere, they often have a silver dagger agenda hidden somewhere.

Or the negative type who is full of drama and negative comments about most things. Both types, from my experience, are extreme cases and big attention seekers and have low self-worth. There is no judgement here, but you must be aware of them as they are...

Total drainers: if you recognise any in your life remove them asap or spend as little time as possible with them. If they are in your family, friendship group or work place this may be difficult, so I strongly suggest you put up really strong boundaries or imagine you have a suit of armour on every time you see them to protect your energy and yourself! They will only cause problems later, especially when you start to move forward.

Their stories and bravado is to boost themselves or cover up what they consider as imperfections in their life, that they don't want others to know about or question. It is all fear-based and the result is that others feel bad and question why their life is not like this. The Pollyanna person feeds off this to make themselves feel better, raise their self-esteem, and try to convince themselves everything is perfect when there is no such thing as perfect.

The negative person wants to bring everyone down to their level and don't you dare try and move forward and be positive. Negative people are quite needy and require lots of love and attention, so much so they are a complete drain. They don't feel good about themselves, which is sad but there is a limit on how many times you can lift them up. If they are not choosing to do so themselves, you must let them go as we all have our limits and they are here to learn too.

It's totally ok not to feel positive every minute of the day. In fact, it's quite normal and also good to speak up when you have a problem or are feeling a bit down or negative.

A problem shared is a problem halved. I usually try to tune into my feelings or the issue, talk it over with a trusted friend, and work my way through it because I may be feeling like this for just today or this whole week. The important thing is to not allow it to build up, and definitely don't bury it. Communication is key!

It's ok if your life, children, family, partner, career are not perfect – life throws us all curve balls at times, it's all part of our learning. Talking it over and finding a solution or adjusting how you're feeling about it is a good thing. After all, we are only human!

Lighten up and don't be too hard on yourself. I always look at Pollyanna people quite differently now and understand they have issues they are not dealing with, and that's ok. Negative people I give very little time to, or just delete them from my life.

The Rushing Syndrome: many, many years ago, I fell for this. I thought I had to feel so busy all the time, filling every minute of every day to keep up the image of being a good mum and wife, overcompensating, and I felt inadequate if I didn't. People like this live with the fear of missing out (FOMO), needing to be needed, fear of rejection, or worrying what people will think if they don't have a full social calendar or they are not busy all the time.

When you have a conversation with them, notice that they often divert the conversation to all about you and your life, giving no time for you to ask too much about them and theirs. They don't stop, think, and feel what they are running from and don't deal well with what others think. My view? They are uncomfortable usually with just *being*.

Do you know people like this or recognise these traits in yourself? It's ok. Remember, awareness is the key to making changes. Stop rushing from one appointment or thing to another. Just allow yourself time and space between to breathe and just *be*.

It's ok to let the fear go and be brave enough to just stop and FEEL!

Gaining awareness is the key, and then you can move through it. Remember, the sun will rise again tomorrow so get back on your bike for a fresh start to a new day

Admitting to your dysfunction is the lesson and it's ok. This gives you the opportunity to move forward, grow, and take steps to change, make better choices, and improve your life.

Yes, we are a product of our past and/or present environment, but that doesn't mean we have to remain a part of it or repeat the genetic history attached to it. We have a **choice to change!**

Don't allow dysfunction of past experiences or anything

you feel you have failed at, keep you stuck where you are or define who you are. Every day you have the opportunity to move forward to a better U.

As I have evolved through my life, people, places and situations have come and gone. I find it easier now to let go of the old, which opens me up to all the new. I let go of genetic and trauma-patterning, past injustices and emotions that have hindered my growth. I now let go of all the hurt around my past learnings and I am now open and ready for the new!

I did it, and it wasn't easy. You have to stick with it, but the results are worth it.

My life is not perfect. I am not perfect and I still work through the lessons, but I now have more balance, peace, happiness, contentment and am grateful for all the awareness. I have a healthier attitude and I feel good about being me.

So flip the attitude to 'It's ok, my life wasn't or isn't perfect', and find a lightness in it.

Gratitude for my dysfunction!

Commit to dedicating a little time for **U** right **now**. Just set up 15 minutes a day to start by setting your phone or a note as a reminder somewhere. This could be early mornings, later in evening, on your lunch break, or all three! If it works, find a regular time that will make it easy to achieve.

Give yourself the **time and strength to be your best** and not anyone else's version! Honour your uniqueness and who you are!

Notice or journal any feelings or things that move for you while you are making changes – it can be very interesting to go back to later!

> *"A healthy attitude is contagious,*
> *but don't wait to catch it from others.*
> *Be a carrier!"*
>
> ~Everyday Health

ACTION

"You're always free to change your mind and choose a different future."

~Richard Bach

Where would I like to change my attitude? Write a list.

. . . .

. . . .

. . . .

How can I work towards achieving this? (Maybe just simply press that delete button in your brain when the negative attitude appears and change it up to a positive one.)

. . . .

. . . .

Write a few positive statements that will flip your previous negatives.

. . . .

. . . .

Be The Best U

Am I rushing too much and cramming too much into every day? Yes or No?

. . . .

Is it out of fear, rejection, not being needed, or what others think?

. . . .

. . . .

Am I projecting to the world that my life is perfect and why?

. . . .

If so, how can I make changes?

. . . .

. . . .

Go get your diary or mobile phone and start now. Mark each month with a change in attitude U can put into action from your list!

ONLY U CAN MAKE IT HAPPEN!

CHAPTER 10

STRESS AND ANXIETY

Stress has become like a badge of honour we all feel we must wear. When we begin to reduce our stress levels, it can feel weird and sometimes uncomfortable, especially if this has been a normal and long-term way of life!

Let go of all the media attachments and just sit with a cup of tea, coffee, or water in the garden, on your deck, in the nearby park, kids' playground, or the beach. Take in what is around you. Leave your phone and iPad in the car, home, or office. Guess what? The world will not end because you're not connected to social media for fifteen minutes.

Breathe in the fresh air, enjoy nature and peace, and really feel it. Your body will start to relax, stress levels will drop, and you will feel more peaceful and re-energised to continue through your day!

OR

It may suit you better to enjoy this at the end of the day while having a bath or going to bed fifteen minutes earlier. Listen to some relaxing music or learn to meditate, which can be just listening to relaxing music or guided meditation. You don't need to do the full yogic thing. Read a real book instead of an e-book, turn the pages, use a beautiful bookmark.

The difference between stress and anxiety

Stress can be a positive thing like meeting a deadline – short term.

Anxiety is constant worrying – longer term.

If short-term stress continues on a regular basis and you don't get a break from it, it can then develop into anxiety and long-term stress – a vicious circle.

So we must give ourselves permission to take that break after any stressful situation and seek help or guidance if needed. Listen to those close to you, as sometimes we cannot see the forest for the trees when we need that break or change.

We are now seeing too many sad results of stress and prolonged anxiety among young people.

"Worrying is praying for something you don't want."

~Anonymous

Resilience is what we need to build within us to cope with the everyday stresses and unexpected issues that may occur. The best way to **grow** our **resilience** so we can **bounce** back from the stresses of life is gained by **reducing stress and improving our sleep.**

Good, restful, deep sleep is how our internal battery recharges. So take some action on how you can improve your sleep to assist your body to build resilience, feel fresh, and re-energised.

Positive affirmation to repeat to yourself daily

'Today, I have all the energy I need. Every cell in my body is now strong, healthy, and full of positive energy.'

Reduce stress by simply practising being in the present moment as often as you can, like if you're stuck in traffic or the supermarket queue – anything that is completely out of your control.

Your unhappiness, anger, and frustration begin to build because your mind takes over. It starts all the chatter because we are not in control of the situation and we have become a very impatient society.

However, if we just **let go and relax** our minds by just **breathing in and out slowly**, then we will start to feel some freedom from our mind's chatter. If we practise this often while having to wait, it will become a healthy habit. Once this becomes a habit, you will begin to notice a change in how you relate to people and situations, and you will **Respond** more than **React**.

Try this

Next time you are in a stressful or frustrating situation, just say to yourself, 'Can I change this situation? Is it out of my control?' Yes, it is!

Now, time to start to breathe slowly and easily from the bottom of your belly all the way up and out. Keep a slow, easy rhythm until you begin to feel more relaxed and less stressed.

Say to yourself, 'This will all pass. Be patient and breathe'. This is practising the present moment. It's that simple, and it's a great exercise to share with family and friends.

"In the midst of movement and chaos, keep stillness inside of you!"

~Deepak Chopra

Multi-skilling creates a lot of stress. We all feel so in control and we are congratulated as a person the more balls we can juggle getting through each day – I know, I've been there! But I've come to realise that **single-skilling** is so much less stressful.

Once you feel tired and over-extended, the buzz starts to disappear from your life. Start designing your own life and routines that suit you and your lifestyle *only* – not what others think or do! Drop things from your life you don't enjoy or hand those things to someone else. Add things you do enjoy and try something new or a better way of doing something.

Over the past ten years, there has been tremendous growth in technology, specifically in mobile phones and the Internet, which we rely on every day for our work and communication. Add the bombardment of Facebook, Instagram, and all social media sites that our bodies and minds aren't built to deal with, and this has an ongoing effect on our health.

Our daily stress levels are affecting us by experiencing poor sleep, having low energy, anxiety, depression, experiencing digestive issues, weight issues, high blood pressure, and adrenal fatigue all from overloading ourselves.

We live so much these days in the fight or flight syndrome, which should only be drawn on when we are in a true fight or flight situation, and not use it as a way of getting through daily life. Living in constant fight or flight puts a lot of pressure on our kidneys and adrenals, that's why there is so much adrenal fatigue and mental health issues diagnosed these days.

"We are sitting under the tree of our thinking minds wondering why we're not getting any sunshine!"

~Ram Dass

The quickest way to slow the body and mind is with long, slow, rhythmic breathing from the belly. **Stop for five minutes and try it**. It may feel weird to start because when we are stressed, we breathe from our upper chest and do short, quick, shallow breathing instead of the long, slow breath drawn from our lower belly.

Breathing long and slow speaks to our nervous system and tells us, 'It's ok, I am safe'.

Change multi-skilling to single-skilling. It brings more focus and clarity and you become more productive and less scattered. Block out time to complete a task with no interruptions from the most major to the most minor tasks at home and at work.

Categorise the tasks, add a timeframe to the block of time, even for 15–30 minutes (or longer depending on the task), complete it, and then move to the next task or block of time. You will feel lighter, clearer, focused, and less stressed.

BE YOUR OWN PERSONAL ASSISTANT BY BLOCKING OUT TIME FOR YOUR TASKS.

Also set yourself a little challenge in this blocked-out time, like completing or reaching the next stage, and then have a short break before moving on to the next task. The break may be some nourishing food, a cuppa, water, stretching and walking around in the fresh air for a few minutes, or just closing your eyes and enjoying some long, slow breathing.

This creates calmness, you will feel accomplished, and it allows more good stuff into your life!

Now...

Clear the clutter and get organised but don't over-organise or you start to micro-manage, which can create stress!

Looking at and working in a messy environment can have you feeling unhappy and overwhelmed with life on all levels. Clutter can make most of us feel anxious, depressed, or even guilty. It can also affect our focus, and our brain's ability to process information. It is stuck-energy and has a huge effect on our lives.

No one likes the thought of spending time clearing stuff and the thought of it can even cause more stress – **mess leads to stress!** Creating order in our lives helps us focus more easily and become more productive at work and at home.

Make it fun and put on some happy music while you clear, and encourage others to join in! You will feel terrific, lighter, happier, and clearer afterwards!

Celebrate after you finish your de-clutter, and make a regular appointment in your diary to keep on top of it. Start your de-clutter list and focus working on one area, one step at a time – not all done in a day. Maybe each day you can spend 10 minutes tidying and de-cluttering your desk at end of the day to give you an organised start the following day. Clear the kitchen at night to have a nice start the next morning.

Have a tub or tray for each person at home where they can put their stuff. At the end of the day/week, they take it and clear it. I know I covered this earlier, but it's a reminder to help with our stress and anxiety levels.

To Do list

- Where do I need to de-clutter often?
- Who can help?

Just gaining a balanced daily routine has a big effect on our daily stress levels.

Organising your week makes your days flow more easily, so put in a little time looking over your week ahead and do a little planning. A little prep time at night sets you up well for the next day, like with your clothes, lunches, snacks, or sports gear – if you share your household, don't forget to delegate.

Plan meals for the week and shop once a week for food. Online shopping saves time.

Do all your personal things like morning walk/run, meditation, and nutritious breakfast before you look at your emails, Facebook, or phones, and make it a house rule.

Getting up 15 minutes earlier each day gives you a great start!

Practise deep, slow breathing, or listen to an app to guide you through meditative breathing. You can also put a note somewhere that you see daily like your work desk, car, phone, or the bathroom.

Just slow down and breathe.

Increase the antioxidants in your food plan. Eat lots of fresh plant-based foods to support your body and a daily antioxidant/immune support supplement if needed. **Greens are your friends.** How do you expect to feel energised and get through your day if you're not eating well?

"Who else wants to shut off their phone, drive to the beach, forget everything, and listen to the sound of the waves crashing?"

~lessons learned life

We all need to be really conscious of simplifying our lives by getting back in touch with nature – the best natural de-stresser. Walk in the mountains, beaches, parks and gardens, try camping. When was the last time you walked through a forest to breathe in the fresh air, touch and feel the energy of the trees?

We all need to learn to Stop, Breathe, and Feel more often.

Take care of stress before it takes care of U!

"We all have a choice. We can agree to live in this culture of stress where we wear stress as a badge of honour or we can say 'No, I'm going to live my life differently!'"

~Dr Lissa Rankin, MD

ACTION

WRITE IT OUT. WHAT CAUSES ME STRESS?

☐ Work . . . .

☐ Family or other relationships . . . .

☐ Finances . . . .

☐ Clutter . . . .

☐ Procrastinating . . . .

☐ Other . . . .

What can I put into action to reduce my stress?

. . . .

. . . .

Where can I take my foot off the peddle?

. . . .

. . . .

If I stop worrying, is the world going to end?

. . . .

Where am I multi-skilling too much?

....

....

How can I change to single-skilling?

....

....

What can I delegate to ease my load?

....

....

Make a De-clutter List, and who can help?

....

....

CHAPTER 11

SOCIAL MEDIA
- CYBER SLAVE

I mentioned under 'Perfection' the negative impact social media is causing in society – adults and teenagers being bullied; children and adults feeling inadequate, losing their self-esteem and self-worth; anxiety; stress; jealousy; competitiveness; suicide; and the growing epidemic of narcissism. I see the results of this in my health studio and it's increasing in adults and children. There are growing mental health issues in young people more than ever before. Social media anxiety is driven by the Fear of Missing Out (FOMO) or what others will think.

"Before you speak, let your words
pass through three gates:
Is it true? Is it necessary? Is it kind?"

~Rumi

Yes, the positive effect of social media is fantastic when it comes to keeping in contact with family and friends, when travelling or moving interstate or overseas. Staying in touch with people in hospital or those who are confined to their homes. It is a real positive when trying to keep in contact with friends, family and the world! Keep in touch and share positive information.

"Adult friendships are hard. Everyone is busy and life happens. I've learned you gotta text people when you're thinking of them. A simple 'Thinking of you, hope all is well' really goes a long way."

~Rob Lowe

However, the real concern now is the overuse and the rubbish we are bombarded with every minute of every day with social media. Putting out information without thinking how some things may affect others, how you see yourself, and how you feel the world sees U. The trolling and abuse towards others is unacceptable behaviour, so sad and very disturbing this is how some in society choose to use it.

There's nothing better than seeing happy, smiling faces doing lots of fun stuff. It's all the selfies, full body shots, food and posts that say, 'I know my real friends will like and share this'.

So I'm no longer a friend if I'm not as active on Facebook (FB), Twitter, Instagram etc? The misinterpretation of comments can also destroy friendships and other relationships. It is very sad and shallow if this is how personal relationships are now judged.

Rethink society. Why are we allowing technology and social media to control and rule our lives ?

Take back your power and control your own life!

We are all unique, extraordinary individuals. However, there's a growing obsession with selfies. Our aesthetic and beauty standards have reached a very high level of expectation. We all need to move, change, respect, and own who we are and what we are about. Think about your energy after you have been on social media – light and happy or the opposite? It only gives me a slight lift when it's a positive!

Social media is sucking the joy out of our lives!

Lack of real communication is the problem as we have all become so self-reliant (myself included) on flicking a text message. It's got its good points when we are all busy. It saves us time in lots of areas such as confirming appointments or answering quickly when you don't have time for a lengthy phone call, and a quick yes or no is needed. A quick text to see how someone you care about is, with a positive message.

However, it is now replacing real communication – the one-on-one, face-to-face conversations. The chat where you can see, feel, express your emotions and receive from the other person. The worst example of this is breaking up a relationship or ending a friendship by email, text or social media. How easy, cold, unemotional, and disrespectful that is to treat another that way. My view is that these people are cowards and unable to deal with real life, up front and honestly.

Jealousy and competitiveness are what social media has assisted to grow. There is no empathy about how this may affect others. It is creating anxiety and depression for those who feel their life is not living up to the social media expectations others are portraying. And I say 'portraying' as most times...

All is never what it appears.

Often, those constantly displaying selfies and everything they do every day or week may actually have low self-esteem and need to use social media to feel good about themselves, to project how wonderful their life is. The amount of friends, likes, and followers they get suggests looking for attention and recognition.

Another stress it creates for those very active on social media, is if someone isn't getting enough likes. What has society come to? Why do we have to display our whole life on social media? And then complain about privacy? We are all adding to the invasion of our privacy.

If you're one of my friends, I'm only on FB occasionally so I would be the worst friend in the world because I choose not to be too active on social media. I respect mine and others' privacy by not participating very often. I don't need my whole life out there for the world to see and comment on as I feel comfortable with who I am and my life.

Some people feel quite inadequate, jealous, depressed, and bored. They ask, 'Why isn't my life like that?' if they have no holiday photos; if they don't go out for dinner, lunch, or coffee all the time; or if it appears they are not having as much fun or have as great a toned body.

Most people constantly posting don't realise the impact it can have on others. It's something you need to think twice about before posting. Take some action and cut back on personal social media accounts and make real contact and communicate with family and friends, or **just get off it** and go for a walk or do something more purposeful, creative, productive.

Another concern is how much time people spend on social media – from dawn until midnight and beyond. Is it boredom or is it the addiction and voyeurism of others' lives we have become attached to?

Too much time on technological devices, I feel, is like pouring fuel into the car and letting it flow out onto the ground, draining our energy.

We have digital detox at our dining table for every meal and we are very conscious of it when we are out. Frustrates our family a little as we don't answer our phones after a certain time at night and most often they are on silent – we choose when and what time we check our phones and messages. It's about respect and being present with who you are with and communicating with each other.

Let go of competitiveness with others – their weight, family, financial situation; how many times they visit the gym, run, or walk; or how many times they eat out a week. Remember to be truly happy being U, just focus on what makes U happy or what sits comfortably with U and your life!

Yes, technology is a necessary part of our lives. Just drop the overuse and think before U post anything!

"Comparison is the thief of joy."

~Theodore Roosevelt

ACTION

ARE YOU A CYBER SLAVE?

If you think you are a slave to social media and other technological devices, you probably are! There are ways to combat this. You can turn off notifications while working on other projects to lessen the distraction, or set time limits for social media.

We all have the choice to shift the world, and we have an obligation to do it from where we stand! Our brains are like batteries. They need to rest and recharge. Stop! Turn off everything to allow your brain and body to recover.

Don't let the digital world control your life! Allocate a social-media-free day every week for you and those around you. Enjoy getting back to you, your surroundings and those you love.

Communicate and focus only on the people, places, and things around you that day. Put all devices away and just check in on phone calls at end of that day – no scrolling your phones – and instead replace it with other activities. It's tough but it does work. Break the addiction because it is slowly damaging your life.

Set up a challenge and throw the challenge out at home and your workplace!

How can I reduce my time on social media each day?

....

Am I suffering from FOMO? If so, why?

....

Do I really need to post as much as I do?

. . . .

Is my energy down after social media?

. . . .

Do I sleep well after?

. . . .

Can I text less and learn to communicate more with family and friends?

. . . .

How can I take control of other media and take digital breaks from emails or blogging? Maybe physically block out times each day to check and deal with these only – this will increase your focus and productivity in other areas.

How can I rest my brain and use this time to do relaxing, mindfulness things?

Just five to ten minutes of slow breaths work. Close your eyes and start breathing from the belly daily – yes, even on your breaks at work. It helps to refresh, relax, and recharge the body and mind. Most importantly, sleep and sleep well!

EMBRACE THE CHALLENGE!

CHAPTER 12

HAPPINESS AND JOY

A state of happiness: A source or cause of delight. A sensation that stems from enjoyment, pleasure, and satisfaction.

Joy is the highest energy of all.

It's that magical feeling that everything is possible. Joy is from appreciating the gifts around us in each moment. When you experience the energy of joy, it allows you to attract and create your present and future moments at their highest possible vibrational level.

What is happiness or what really makes U happy?

Happiness comes from within. It is different for everyone!

Happiness is simple. We live in a society that feeds on stress. In fact, a lot of us have accepted high levels of stress to be normal, wearing it like a badge of honour and yet stress is our biggest killer. It creates 'dis-ease' in our bodies.

It's expected for us all to walk around daily saying, 'I'm really busy and stressed' as if it's abnormal if you say: 'I'm really good and having a great day'. People sometimes look at you like you're weird. Or are they secretly thinking, *How can they say that? Why are they not stressed? How can they be relaxed?* or *I'd like what he/she is having!* So choose now if you want a happier, healthier life, and start simply but consistently to achieve visiting your happy place on a daily basis – where there is no stress!

We are all in search of happiness. It's up to U to find it!

"Happiness is like a butterfly which, when pursued, is always beyond our grasp, but if you will sit down quietly, may alight upon you."

~Nathaniel Hawthorne

Find Your Happy Place!

Here is an article that a close and brave friend of mine wrote. This is what I'm talking about. Why do we wait for the wake-up call before we try and find our happy place? Learn from this personal story.

"It was There all the Time, a Place of Peace."

~Trish Lawrence

Three months ago, I was thrown a curve ball by being told I had a rare melanoma. And with all that has happened since, I have certainly learned to see life through different eyes.

I have found my happy place and I didn't have to go far. It is my front garden in the beautiful coastal town where I live. Our raised block sits amongst the most beautiful and majestic Moonah trees. I sit on our deck in the shadows of these tall and shapely timbers and take it all in.

We have a bird bath that brings in the wattle birds, magpies, and blackbirds. There can sometimes be a queue waiting their turn for a bath. I can hear the roar of the ocean and the songs of the birds around me. The magpies tell me their story, and the sound is so Australian.

When I look up through the Moonahs, I am always amazed at the different shapes they make. They reach out to hold each other up. At night, they become quite ghostly and take on a whole different picture. I never get sick of looking at them.

My Thai Buddha sits comfortably in the garden among the native grasses and a huge bird's nest fern. He is a constant reminder that to find peace, you have to reach into your mind and be with it in your 'special place'.

Sometimes, a curve ball is not such a bad thing. You learn to play a different game.

♡

Unfortunately, after eighteen months of being clear, the melanoma returned aggressively to take her away from her happy place very quickly, just when I was close to finishing this book. You were an amazing, happy woman who put up a brave fight, kept smiling, and opened your heart to all the love and support around you. You're now resting, my friend, in another world of love and peace, your new happy place.

♡

Why do we wait? Why does happiness and peace elude us? Because we say, 'I'll just get this', 'reach this achievement'… But all the money in the world cannot save us from the inevitable.

However, we delay finding peace and happiness. We can still have our material things, but we all need to find our happy place, even for just fifteen minutes a day. This is what mindfulness is – just sitting, appreciating, being grateful, and taking in the world around us.

This one crazy, beautiful life we are here to enjoy. For however long, we do not know!

"None of us are getting out of here alive, so please stop treating yourself like an afterthought. Eat the delicious food, walk in the sunshine, jump in the ocean. Say the truth that you're carrying in your heart like a hidden treasure. Be silly, be kind, be weird. There's no time for anything else."

~Richard Gere

My Happy Place

None of us has to search for happiness. It's usually simple and right in front of us!

Mine is a lovely beach walk or through our beautiful park overlooking the bay, where my children played many years before. It's the memories of taking a drink and snacks while watching them play, shared with friends and family.

The happy times swimming and surfing at the beach; cheering them on at their sporting events and shared with other parents and the community. We were all happy supporting each other for one purpose: our children.

Now that they are adults, it's observing them around our large dining table with their partners and sometimes friends just chatting, catching up, laughing, and enjoying a meal and a glass of wine together.

In those moments, I stand in my kitchen and soak in what I see, hear, and feel: the noise of the happy energy those moments bring. They can be fleeting, so I like to stop, listen, and catch those moments when I can.

Now, playing with my grandchildren, sitting on the floor and building their favourite train set together. Playing ball, running around my garden, their laughter when Nanna does something silly is pure joy! Sharing a meal of their favourites cooked by Nanna and catching up on all their news. Then winding down, sitting in my cosy lounge playing a card game or reading their dad's old favourite books to them, as I did with their dad's when they were young is an absolute blessing. Such special, happy little souls.

Gathering with friends at home for a social catch up, sharing stories and lots of laughs over a good meal and glass of wine.

Starting my day with ten minutes of guided meditation or five – ten minutes of Qigong in the garden, breathing in the clean, fresh air.

Sitting on my deck surrounded by the beautiful natural native garden I created, with the help of my son, his machinery and our joint vision is now a very peaceful place to sit with a cuppa and soak in nature.

It's feeling the light breeze on my face, taking in the stillness of a cold, early morning; the rain and the warm sunshine; watching the clouds float by; the sunrise or sunset; the change of seasons; all the birds flying from tree to tree; and the bees and butterflies pollinating the flowering plants and vegetable garden. I look to see how many I can spot and really listen to the bird life – how many birds I can identify just by their sound. It's standing out under the moon and stars for a few minutes in the evenings and being amazed by the beauty above.

I love to happy dance by myself to my fav music - releases stress, lifts my energy and lights up my brain. Sitting at the beach closing my eyes and listening to the waves lapping at the shore always brings me peace and gratitude.

These are my everyday happy place rituals in just a few minutes to find Balance and Peace in a busy world!

"Happiness is having someone to love, something to do, and something to look forward to."

~Anonymous

"If it is to be, it's up to me!"

~Anonymous

This quote was up on my boys' study desks all through their secondary school years to remind them they could achieve their goals and dreams if they put in the effort. No one just hands it to you on a plate. You need to consistently work towards your dreams and goals or results for a happier life, and I'm proud to say they have all achieved this. They are all now amazing men we are very proud of, very social media/phone conscious and now educating their children to do the same!

Fifteen minutes a day of doing what makes U happy!

What are you going to do with your fifteen minutes? Choose the healthy option for lunch, sit quietly, eat slowly and enjoy. Exercise, walk in nature, and truly take in your surroundings?

No phones or social media allowed during your fifteen minutes.

Read a real book on self-help or a favourite interest. Dance to your favourite music, find something that gives you a calming and uplifting vibe. Just sit and enjoy breathing long and slowly. Stretch!

It may suit you to walk twice a week or blend a few different types of exercise or happy times – variety is the spice of life!

I can't make happiness happen for you. It's something different for everyone. You need to choose whatever it means to you and then take **action** and the necessary steps towards making it happen!

I challenge YOU to dig deep and find what really makes you feel happy and comfortable in your own skin on all levels of your life... and do it!

ACTION

WHATEVER MOVEMENT MAKES U HAPPY – CHOOSE IT AND DO IT!

Go on. The challenge is set. Make a regular 15-minute happy date with yourself daily! Please don't beat yourself up if you miss a day. If it's easier, start once or twice a week and grow from there until it builds into a daily practise.

What really makes me happy? Close your eyes, visualise what is happy to U, and really feel what that is like. What feelings came up?

. . . .

. . . .

. . . .

What is happiness to U? . . . .

. . . .

Where in your body did you feel it? . . . .

. . . .

When was the last time, if at all, you felt this happiness?

. . . .

What action steps can you start to take to achieve this feeling of happiness for U?

. . . .

When, where, and what will I do on my happiness date with me?

. . . .

Take responsibility
for your own happiness!

"To blame another for our misfortunes shows lack of education. To blame oneself for one's misfortunes shows your education has begun. When you blame no one, your education is complete."

~Bruce Lipton – *Biology of Belief*

CHAPTER 13

CLEAR THE CLUTTER IN YOUR LIFE!

Yes, that means your home, workspace, wardrobe, and all the stuff we hoard as humans!

Clutter is stuck energy. Clearing your spaces helps clear your life!

You will become clearer in your thoughts and have greater focus and clarity in all areas of your life, including relationships.

Feel the joy after clearing the clutter. It's a great feeling and it assists in reducing stress and improving your health and happiness. So go on, be brave, and plan a weekend – or maybe a few, depending on your clutter – or dedicate one day or few hours each week clearing one space at a time until all the clutter is gone.

Tips on how to start:

· Make a list of areas you need to clear, then number them in the order you would like to tackle them. Remember, it doesn't all have to be done in a day, just one job/area at a time. Once you get started, the momentum will grow as you start to feel clearer and more focused.

· Start piles such as 'Op Shop' and 'Tip'. Shred, burn or can I sell it?

· Don't revisit the piles.

· Once you have a boot load for the Op Shop, drop it off for someone else to love.

· Same with the tip, burning, or shredding – just do it!

· Set up an ebay or local Facebook selling page and make a few $$$.

· Leave things on your nature strip to give away or you may have a hard rubbish pick up in your area. You know what they say: 'One man's rubbish is another man's treasure'. If not taken in a week, remove it from the nature strip and drop off where you need to (tip, etc.).

· If you're unsure or you struggle to move things on, hold the garment, article, or piece, close your eyes and feel. Does this lift your energy or deplete it?

Lift - keep.
Deplete - Delete.

- Check in: when did I last use this item? If not in the last twelve months, let it go! What's the worst thing that can happen if you ever need it again? You can buy another.

- Include your tech devices, old emails, text messages, old contacts, receipts, accounts etc.

- Clearing out the old allows you to bring in new energy and a lighter vibe!

- Have fun. Friends or family can help by joining in. Have a declutter BBQ to celebrate. High fives all around!

- Embrace and enjoy the joy of clearing stuck energy. Do a happy dance!

DO YOU WANT TO FEEL HAPPY AND FREE?

"Let go of what's gone, be grateful for what remains, and really look forward to what's coming."

~power positivity

CHAPTER 14

HEALTH AND WELL-BEING

"The secret to living well and longer is eat half, walk double, laugh triple, and love without measure."

~Tibetan proverb

Start with practising self-care for better health and wellness. Dis-ease begins when the body is out of balance. The choices you make each day give you the opportunity to change and give your body the chance to feel well and begin its natural power to heal from within.

A happy heart is a healthy heart, and the same goes for the rest of your body and health – really, it's not that hard. So much information is now available on health, latest diet fads, what's good, and what's not. It's a mine field for the average person to work out, and we all want that quick fix when it comes to weight loss and fitness programmes. Here is a simple way to start looking at your health, food plans, and exercise!

Note: I call it food plan because the minute you say diet, the brain and body go into meltdown, and it means instant restriction. *Oh, I really want all those things I can't have.* Sound familiar?

Well, here's my own simple take on a healthy lifestyle – love it or leave it, your choice. It is only a guide, so feel free to create your own. Always seek medical advice before making changes, especially if you have any pre-existing health issues.

- Check out the healthy weight range for your height.
- Aim for losing 1kg a week if you're overweight.
- Best to stay away from the scales daily as it plays with your mind. Weigh and measure yourself (chest, waist, hips) at the start of your changes, and then again once a month. You can usually gauge the results by your clothes getting looser, which always makes you feel good.
- Five servings of fresh veggies/salad and two pieces of fresh fruit per day. If you need, Google what that looks like.
- Example of portion sizes for veggies (five servings per day):

½ cup cooked green or orange veggies (zucchini, carrot, pumpkin, broccoli);

⅔ cup florets cauliflower;

½ cucumber;

¾ cup mushrooms or asparagus spears;

1 cup raw, leafy salad greens and raw salad veggies;

1 tomato;

½ cup sweet corn or small corn cob;

½ medium potato or sweet potato;

½ cup cooked, dried, or canned beans, peas or lentils.

- Example portion sizes of fruit (two servings per day):

  1 medium apple, banana, orange, or pear;

  2 small apricots, kiwifruit, or plums;

  1 cup of diced fruit.

ACTION

Here's a simple guide with ideas to get you started. Enjoy!

Start your day with a good stretch and sip 1 cup of warm water infused with a slice of lemon to kick-start digestion.

BREAKFAST

Banana or other fresh fruit – eaten on its own is better for digestion.

Make a green or berry smoothie the night before to drink if you're on the run. Drink slowly.

Cereal or Bircher muesli made night before with Linseed, Sunflower seeds and Almonds finely ground together (health food aisle) great little boost to blend or sprinkle onto anything, add to yoghurt OR eggs and spinach on toast, baked beans on toast OR avocado on toast. Tea/coffee.

MORNING TEA

Piece of fruit or protein ball. Tea, herbal tea or warm water with lemon.

LUNCH

Mixed salad bowl with either tuna, salmon, chicken or an egg, or in a sandwich, wrap or roll. Soups or bone broth in colder months with lots of veggies plus bread or dry biscuits.

Be The Best U

AFTERNOON SNACK

Apple and nuts; yoghurt; protein ball; hummus dip and veggie sticks; or cheese and biscuits. Tea/water or bone broth in winter.

DINNER

Variety of yellow, orange, and green veggies; sweet potato or small potato with a lean meat, fish or chicken dinner;

DESSERT

Chia pudding, sorbet, fresh berries, stewed fruits of the season, or one piece of dark chocolate with a calming herbal tea.

Drink lots of water daily and save the glass of wine for the weekends to enjoy!

It's important to mix it up for variety. Don't eat the same breakfast every day so it doesn't become boring to you or your body. Break the routine – choose two or three different breakfast menus and swap them around for flexibility. Try this with each meal. Doing this will also assist with you being more flexible in life. We sometimes get a little stuck in our daily routines so change it up!

- Eggs; lots of mixed greens (raw and cooked); basmati or brown rice; fresh fish, chicken, and lean red meat; legumes. There are plenty of recipes and help on the Internet. Breads: spelt, rye, or multi-grain if you need extra fibre. Gluten-free if needed.

- Protein and carbs create fuel for our body so make sure you have a nice balance of these daily. A boost of real food protein to drink after exercise aids recovery.

- Gut health is really important as our gut is now known as our second brain. Did you know that lots of happy hormones are made in the gut then sent to the brain? Besides all the other amazing work the gut does, it's so important for it to be healthy. Our gut is hugely affected by stress and how we are emotionally digesting life or what is eating away at U!
Seek advice for a happy gut.

- Water: keep a bottle in your car, on your desk, and jug on the bench at home. Drink tea, herbal tea and limit coffee.

- Choose foods that are grilled, barbecued, steamed, or poached. Choose tomato-based sauces, or teriyaki and vinaigrette sauces in place of creamy ones. Try olive oil and lemon juice with a dash of apple cider vinegar or seedy mustard as a dressing.

- Portion plates are now available to help understand portion sizes. Good idea is to split your plate into three: fill half your plate with salad or vegies then ¼ with low to medium GI Carbs, ¼ with lean proteins. Only use this as a general guide as the amount of energy you need daily may vary pending exercise, physical activity etc. Seek personalised support from an accredited dietitian for advice.

- Eat an 80% alkaline and 20% acid food intake. Our bodies need a good alkaline reading to support the body's natural ability to fight dis-ease. Google up the info or pop into your health food store for advice and buy some PH strips to test your alkaline levels regularly.

Create a rainbow of colour on your plate every meal and enjoy!

Go easy on:

- Alcohol – try and avoid alcohol during the week and enjoy a glass on the weekend.
- Butter or margarine – keep to a minimum or use avocado, hummus as alternatives.
- Coconut products.
- Breads and bread products.

Avoid:

- Sugar – our biggest problem.
- Sports drinks and soft drinks – high in sugar and salt.
- Fried foods.
- Creamy sauces, mayonnaise, creamy cheeses.
- Pesto – can be very oily.
- Pastries and cakes.

Remember that this is only a few of my personal ideas. To assist you in creating your own personal food plan and adjusting around any health issues, allergies, exercise or other health requirements, seek advice from a nutritionist or a dietician.

Organising tips

- Plan ahead for the week. It takes a few minutes to Meal Plan. Write down what you need to buy for breakfast, lunch and dinner for the week.

- Spend some time buying, washing, chopping, or cutting salad/veggies into containers to prepare them to make your delish meals.

- Prepare lunches or smoothies the night before, if possible, to help with busy mornings.

- Always have a lovely bowl of fruits of the season and a container of nuts and dips nearby to snack on.

Little effort for a great result!

- If you miss a few days or over-indulge, don't beat yourself up. Forgive yourself, put it behind you, and start again the next day!

- If your food and exercise is balanced consistently, you can have those cheat days and recover. After all, we need to enjoy life as well!

Start now

Make simple, consistent changes so that they become a healthy habit for a healthier life!

"Every day is a new beginning.
Take a deep breath and start again."

~Anonymous

CHAPTER 15

ENERGY IN
- ENERGY OUT!

Remember that fresh foods supply your body with energy. When you move, you use energy. If you eat more than the calories you burn, you will gain those kilos and vice versa. It is that simple.

Kilos can slowly be gained. A few grams a week add up to a few kilos a year, and in a few years, many kilos can be gained.

Increasing your energy output and making a few healthy adjustments to your daily food plan will give positive results!

Exercise helps to burn body fat, increase muscle, reduce digestive issues, improve your immune system, increase bone strength, calm our brain and raise endorphin levels to make you feel happier!

Just 15–30 minutes a day of exercise three times a week will help to reduce weight, improve fitness, reduce stress and clear your mind. This only needs to be a quick-paced walk around the block to start, and then longer as you feel more energised. You can also try yoga, go to the gym, or join dance sessions if you like. Try the Internet for exercising at home.

Use your lunchbreak as exercise time by taking the stairs,

or park your car a little further from work and walk the rest of the way. Add extra time over the weekend to make it fun and not a chore. Rediscover your surroundings. Plan a different walk or bike ride each weekend.

Did you know that scientific research has shown the health benefits of a Zumba class compared to a Tai Chi class are exactly the same to your body – how amazing!

Meet a friend for coffee or lunch, park the car a good distance away and walk there and back. Walk the dog and breathe in that fresh air. It doesn't need to be boot camp and you don't need to pay expensive gym fees. However, if you enjoy the gym and work under the guidance of personal trainers, then that's great – whatever works for you and your lifestyle!

Create a personal plan that works for U and your body!

Keep hydrated every day. Keep a water bottle on your desk at work, in the car, or on the kitchen bench to remind you to drink more water! Adding some slices of lemon makes the water taste better, plus it's good for you, and aids digestion.

Watch your wee and keep it clear!
Check and Detect your bowel!

- If your urine is clear to a pale straw colour, you're hydrated.

- Bright yellow colour could be from taking vitamins but it may also mean that you need to up your water intake.

- Light green to gold colour may mean dehydration is occurring and you should up your water intake immediately.

- Darker brown colour may mean severe dehydration so drink lots water ASAP and consistently. This can also occur if you have just completed heavy exercise training, so electrolytes may also be helpful.

- Darker colour that stays frothy regularly means you need to get to your GP as it may indicate a health issue.

- Keep an eye on your wee every time you pee because it's a good natural indicator of your hydration levels. Remember that the body is made up of 70% water so it makes sense to keep hydrated.

- Also be very aware of any bowel changes or digestive issues, blood in your stools or on toilet paper, bloating, pain, unusual reflux or indigestion. Seek medical advice no matter your age as there is a high percentage of bowel cancer detected in under-50s and now rising in those aged 25-29 years. It is no longer an old person's disease, and in many cases if diagnosed early, the greater the success rate. Check, Detect and seek medical advice if needed!

CHAPTER 16

WELLNESS TIPS

- Start with a great attitude – it's great to be alive.

- Every day is a new day – be aware of how lucky you are.

- Stop blaming others for your choices – be responsible for your choices to exercise, eat healthy and improve your life.

- Avoid toxic, draining people and attitudes – they will bring you down.

- Eat healthy and aim to keep your body alkaline by eating 80% alkaline and 20% neutral or 'acid' foods (Google) – strengthens our bodies to fight dis-ease.

- Be aware of any physical or health restrictions – work around them and do what you can.

- Eliminate the stress – stop sweating the small stuff and just let go.

- Stop comparing yourself to others – remind yourself that you love U as the unique person U are

- 'I can' attitude – practise this no matter what.

- Age is no barrier – enjoy each year and celebrate each special decade.

- Celebrate the day you arrived here – it's your own special birth-day! Buy yourself a gift and if you can't celebrate with others or even one person, go do something nice for U!

- Learn something new – add a new activity each year.

- Give back a little with volunteer work – assists you to have gratitude for your own life and it beats sitting at home and being lonely.

- Enjoy your community and the area where you live – discover it like a tourist.

- Embrace close family and friends – they are gold.

- Be happy – find your happy place and be there as often as you can.

- You are No. 1! So live your life well for U!

"My true self leads me to an inspired life."

~Deepak Chopra

Note: more wellness tips and guidance available in my booklet *Wellness with the Seasons* eat and move your body with the four seasons – available through most Internet bookstores.

CHAPTER 17

RELATIONSHIPS

"There are four very important words in life: love, honesty, truth, and respect. Without these in your life, you have nothing."

~power positivity

Relationships are never easy and are always a work in progress. Sometimes, they flow easily; other times, they are quite challenging. We need to keep growing and learning as a person, which has a knock-on effect on all our relationships.

My rule of thumb:

"People are in your life for a reason, season, or a lifetime."

~Anonymous

Very few people are there for a lifetime. When you look at it this way, it's fascinating which category they fall into and how much learning you gain from this outlook.

People drift in and out of our lives over a lifetime, some briefly, and others for much longer. There is a blend of love, happiness, and learning with all of them. However, the more we grow, the more some of these relationships may be challenged.

Never be afraid of this because it shows us that we are learning and moving forward. Maybe we outgrow some of them and vice versa. While it can be sad when you lose a friend, a partner, or a relative, there are always more people who will come along to enrich your life.

ENJOY THEM ALL FOR THE LOVE, HAPPINESS, GROWTH, AND LEARNING THEY BRING!

· **Love** yourself first, and it will shine out to others – open your heart.

· **Honesty** is the best policy – practise honesty, it builds trust.

· **Truth** goes with honesty – if there is lack of either of these, it needs to be addressed. Communicate and discuss openly where there needs to be more truth and honesty, and determine why it is happening – old habits, conditioning, situation, issues or events that have contributed. Afterward, decide on the best way to openly discuss ways to improve the issue. And it's ok if you need professional help for guidance.

· **Respect** like love begins with respecting U first, and you deserve respect from others. Like they deserve respect from U.

If I could believe one positive thing about me, what would it be?

What are the positive aspects of the most important people and relationships in your life? Remember that none of us are perfect! Learn to respect U and others. Ask yourself what is it you need to know more of and understand about yourself, the people around you, and your close relationships.

Communication is the key in life!

If you don't communicate in a healthy way how you are feeling or the affect it may be having on you, how can you expect someone else to read your mind and understand? It's a two-way street of understanding each other.

Note: Tony Robbins has some great info on YouTube about personal relationships, their challenges, breakdowns, and repairs. It's worth a look, and even better if you can share it with the other person you are in conflict with. This may be a good alternative if one or both parties are a little reluctant to seek professional help.

ACTION

Remember that none of us are perfect, but we all deserve to be truly loved and respected!

Are you being true to you and your relationships?

. . . .

Are there any negative people in your life at the moment? Who are they?

. . . .

How do they make you feel?

. . . .

How much time do you need to spend with them?

. . . .

Who are the most important people/relationships in your life now and write their most positive aspects next to their names.

. . . .

What is it you need to understand more about yourself in your close relationships?

. . . .

How are you as a friend and partner?

. . . .

Do you need to make any changes to your attitude or how you react/respond?

....

If you need to give more in your relationships – how?

....

What more would you like to receive from your relationships?

....

How do you deserve to be treated?

....

How should you be treating others with...

....

Is there any more you need to give in any of your relationships? Or are you giving too much and need to step back and create some boundaries for yourself?

....

....

What are the boundaries?

....

Notice the good
in others and genuinely
thank them for any
kind gestures.

CELEBRATE OTHERS' VICTORIES OR ACHIEVEMENTS - DROP THE JEALOUSY.

CHAPTER 18

FORGIVENESS!

Forgiveness is the nuts and bolts of where we need to start to improve all our relationships.

"Holding on to anger and resentment is like drinking poison and expecting the other person to die."

~Buddha

Once you recognise your past negative emotions such as anger, fear, guilt, anxiety, and sadness...

Write them down so you can then let them go!

This is my process of a full-moon ritual I do each month. I write a forgiveness letter of any incident, trauma, person, place, or thing that has hurt me over the years (or presently) and how it made me feel. Then I safely burn the letter outside under the moon, releasing it to leave in the care of the universal post office. Putting pen to paper with words allows the mind, body, and spirit to heal.

Sometimes, this can be a difficult letter to write, and we may not know where to start. Please put U as the first person on your list to forgive, and then continue with the rest. If you are unsure how to begin, you can just simply forgive yourself on the first full moon or use this example below instead.

Formula for forgiveness by Charles Fillmore

"I forgive everything, everyone, every experience, every memory of the past or present that needs forgiveness. I forgive positively everyone. I also forgive myself of past mistakes.

The universe is love and I am forgiven and governed by love alone. Love is now adjusting my life. Realising this, I abide in peace!"

Write it down, read it, feel it, and then burn it safely to the universe. I do all four – write, read, feel and speak it – then burn it safely outside or in your fireplace.

It is a beautiful ritual that will bring you great peace as you do this each month. Sometimes, you may need to repeat the same forgiveness for certain incidents or people if there has been a deep, traumatic hurt until you eventually feel relief. There may be tears or anger, or a mix of both, but those emotions go along with letting go and releasing them from the body so that you can move forward.

AT THE BOTTOM OF THE FORGIVENESS LETTER, I WRITE THAT I OPEN MY HEART AND SEND LOVE TO EVERYONE ON MY LIST!

Sending love to someone who has hurt you is a tough one, but it is the best thing you can do. It assists to break the karmic attachment between you and the person or issue.

This is why you may need to forgive the same people, issues, or yourself a few times and remember to send love. Do this each full moon until you feel peace and resolution. It may just happen the first time or can take a few moons.

It's a form of detachment, and the more you can release and detach, the more you will become the observer of your life. This allows you to look from the outside in and choose to respond better for your highest good in the future with any issues and with others.

Remember, forgiving someone or an issue doesn't mean you have *forgotten* the issue, we need to be aware of it so it doesn't happen to us again. Forgiving is releasing it and letting go of the emotions attached to it, moving it out of your life.

This can be quite a challenging exercise, but you will gain peace. No one needs to know you are doing it and the energetic ripple-effect will spread to others and the issues. The more forgiveness and peace you gain, the better your life will be. It is really nice to let go, forgive, release and move on from old stuff!

FORGIVE THEM, AND MOST IMPORTANTLY, FORGIVE U.

CHAPTER 19

GRATITUDE

"The best way to appreciate someone or something is to imagine your life without them."

~power positivity

Gratitude costs nothing and everyone can easily be grateful for their lives every day. Material success is not as important as the happiness and peace of being grateful for the simple things in life. Gratitude has a positive effect on our brain, emotions, health, relationships, and careers. You also become less materialistic and competitive, more confident, feel more positive, and sleep better.

"Feeling gratitude and not expressing it is like wrapping a present and not giving it."

~William Arthur Ward

Practising gratitude daily for a few minutes when you first wake and just before you fall asleep creates a good, positive habit that just becomes an easy and natural part of your day. Just wake up, stretch, and be grateful that you're alive – that's a great start! If you like journaling, have a small notepad by your bed and write at the beginning and end of your day for a month (or longer if you wish). Before long, you will experience gratitude easily every day and you will feel happier and more positive.

Really think about the farmer who grows our crops, cattle, sheep, chickens and their eggs. The fisherman who risks the great seas to catch our fish. The production line of people who bring the food to the stores and the people who stock the shelves and sell it to us. The fresh water readily available to us and the clean air we breathe. The sunshine and rain and all the benefits they bring. Our health, families, friends, homes, careers, lifestyle... the list goes on.

Maybe just before you eat each meal, have a quiet ritual in your mind, be grateful, and bless the food we eat that keeps us healthy and well.

Putting gratitude into a physical practise is also important, like speaking with gratitude to someone and not just saying thank you. Instead, say something like, 'Thank you for being a kind supportive friend', 'Thank you for cooking this delish dinner for us to enjoy', 'Thanks for bathing the kids and walking the dog. It meant a lot to me'. Let this flow over into your workplace as well.

"Acknowledge the good you already have in your life. It is the foundation for all abundance."

~Eckhart Tolle

Under the full moon each month, after writing your forgiveness letter, write a gratitude letter of every person, place, or thing you are grateful for including yourself. Burn this safely, offering it to the universe, and truly feel grateful as you watch it burn!

After many years of this process every full moon, my forgiveness letter is quite short now and my gratitude letter is very long. I feel peace every time, but it took a while, so be patient with yourself.

Set this time aside each month. You can Google full moon dates and times, then mark them in your diary. Make notes during that day, then write your letter and complete this ritual in the evening before bed.

Forgiveness assists us to move forward, and the more we can open our hearts to forgiveness, love and gratitude, and unblock our stuck areas, the easier change will happen in our lives!

The more we release, the more space there is for good to flow into our lives!

Don't just wait for the full moon before you feel grateful. Make your own ritual of having gratitude every day, just for a moment or two – it really does make you appreciate all we have and brings a calming effect to your life, even just for those few precious moments.

ACTION

ON THE FULL MOON

This can be your own personal and private ritual, or you can have others join in on the forgiveness and gratitude.

· Me – do I need to forgive myself for any mistakes or issues in my life and stop beating myself up?

· Which relationship issues do I need to forgive and let go?

· Others – who do I need to forgive? Are there any issues others created that I need to forgive and let go? How did it make me feel?

Wait for the full moon and write your Forgiveness Letter – forgive yourself first before forgiving other people, places, traumas, and mistakes. You can also use the 'Forgiveness Formula' under the Forgiveness section – it works!

After you're done, read and feel, then burn safely outside. It can also be fun to note to yourself how it burns. I discovered over the years that the issues or hardest people I need to forgive, burn slowly. Sometimes, I may even have to relight them, while others can burn really fast!

Write and burn your Gratitude Letter – everything you are totally grateful for, even down to the farmer who grows our food, to our warm homes, our family, friends, the fresh water, the air we breathe every day, our health, fitness, and the little changes we make for a better life.

"Dwelling on past bad decisions you have made only allows those decisions to keep defining you. Forgive yourself and move on."

~Mandy Hale – *Simple Reminders*

**Enjoy writing this list.
It is a mindfulness exercise,
and feel the joy of being truly grateful!**

THEN...

ON THE NEW MOON

Write your new moon list of wishes or goals/results you would like to achieve in the coming month. We have an opportunity to do this every month!

Write next to each one, the steps you can take to support achieving it and how you will feel when you do achieve this. Make sure to really feel the emotion. Play with the list, make it vibrant and fun! You can incorporate colour, images, drawings, and positive words, then pin it up somewhere you can read often during the month like inside your wardrobe door.

When the next new moon comes around, check off from the list how many things you achieved. You may just want to aim for one thing each month and that's great. Don't beat yourself up if you don't reach all the wishes or goals/results you listed – you can just start again next new moon!

"Be thankful of how rich you really are.
Your family and friends are priceless.
Your time is gold and your
health is your wealth."

~power positivity

CHAPTER 20

LEARNING LIFE LESSONS

I could write hundreds of books on the lessons I have learnt and am still learning, and I hope to never stop learning as this is how we grow and evolve as a person!

"The most important point is to accept yourself and stand on your own two feet. Enjoy your problems."

~Japanese philosophy

Look at your problems as an opportunity. You never see it as such at the time when the problem arises, but if you recognise the learning, growth, and transformation, you will look back and go *aha!* That's why I was gifted that problem.

They don't always have to be big problems either. Smaller issues give us the opportunity to gain perspective and see things in a different light. Learn from everything that comes across your path.

We learn most when we are out of our comfort zone, so don't hide from the discomfort because that's where you experience real growth. This is the part in any problem or situation where I always say to myself:

OK, I DIDN'T LIKE THAT SITUATION, BUT WHAT WAS MY LESSON?

Ask yourself what you needed to learn from the situation. Do you need to stand up for yourself, speak up, listen to others more, be kinder, patient, stop controlling/ manipulating, let go, fearful of having a go, feel more confident, believe in myself, de-stress, chill, lighten up, slow down?

You feel lighter once you recognise the gift of the lesson, and you will move on more quickly instead of holding onto it and storing anger and frustration in your body. Don't worry about others involved in the issue as they also have a lesson to learn – just focus on U!

Learn, let go, and be grateful!

Anything that annoys you is teaching you patience.

Anyone who abandons you is teaching you how to stand on your own two feet.

Anything that angers you is teaching you forgiveness and compassion.

Anything that has power over you is teaching you how to take your power back.

Anything you hate is teaching you
unconditional love.

Anything you fear is teaching you courage
to overcome your fear.

Anything you can't control is teaching you
how to let go!

*"If you're not learning something in this life,
you might as well be dead."*

~Quote from my awesome and wise grandfather, Jack.
Thank you, Pop. I'm still learning!

CHAPTER 21

TRANSFORMATION

Meaning: a marked change in form, nature, or appearance.

As humans, our lives are constantly transforming. The greatest challenge life has to offer is to become true to your inner-self! This means finding greater meaning and satisfaction in what you do on a daily basis. Transformation does not mean sitting on top of a mountain and meditating for the rest of our lives. It means creating and moving inwards to find who we really are, what we want from life, and having a purpose.

"Let difficulty transform you. And it will.
In my experience, we just need help in learning
how not to run away."

~Pema Chodron

We all feel vulnerable and scared at times, usually we hold back because we are fearful of failure, being hurt, rejected, disappointed. We need to risk opening up, saying yes and being more receptive.

Your breakthrough will happen when the pain to stay closed tight as a bud is so great, you will allow yourself to open up and bloom like a beautiful flower.

This can lead us to all sorts of transformation:

· Looking and feeling fitter and healthier.

· Educating ourselves – working towards changing careers, new interests or hobby.

· Travelling and reading to grow our interests and experiences.

· Taking on creative projects.

· Learning more about ourselves, which can transform our personal relationships.

· Gaining greater meaning in our lives and work.

· Working through your fear barriers.

· Reaching out and transforming another life within your community or field. It's about sharing your gifts to assist others, either adults, teenagers or children, to find a better way of life, guiding them to greater confidence and belief in themselves.

· Appreciating nature, which is a beautiful reminder of constant transformation.

Reflect on nature

Rainbows appear after the rain, ugly ducklings always turn into beautiful swans, and caterpillars grow into butterflies. The lotus flower struggles from the muddy water to bloom into a beautiful flower. All of these are reminders that hardship results in positive transformation.

I love the butterfly. In fact, I really love the special blue butterfly and the story of how they begin as a caterpillar cocooning in the darkness. It is the struggle of shedding the cocoon that makes the butterfly's wings strong enough to fly.

It is the tragedy that to become a butterfly, the caterpillar has to fall apart, until just the essence of its former-self is left behind, and it can emerge to the world as a beautiful butterfly!

"Just when the caterpillar thought the world was over, it became a beautiful butterfly."

~dailyquotes.com

Good always comes from adversity.

EMBRACE YOUR TRANSFORMATION

CHAPTER 22

GRIEF

"It takes strength to make your way through grief, to grab hold of life and let it pull you forward."

~Patti Davis

Grief is a part of life that is not just connected to death. It is any form of loss – career, people, pets, relationship, home, or friendship.

It's ok to grieve. In fact, it is healthy to just let out how we are feeling, expressing how it is making us feel inside, and letting the tears flow. It's a good, positive thing to assist in relieving grief – letting it out. It's ok not to be strong all the time and learn to be a little vulnerable and lean on those who love and support you instead.

Sometimes we need professional help to guide us through, especially if the loss has left a big hole in our lives. Grief and loss are unavoidable during our lifetime, and how we process what happened is different for each of us.

The loss of a loved one never really leaves us, but the pain does ease and soften over time. We usually have beautiful memories to help ease that pain.

I have personally experienced most forms of death throughout my life, and one particular year I lost three people very close to me within ten days. I can't even put into words the pain I experienced then. However, it became a transformational time in my life, and it completely changed my perspective on death and loss, after much grieving and soul searching.

We all need lots of support, love, and understanding at any time that we experience loss. However, we must also remember not to become a victim to the sadness because this can cause us to go into a sadder, deeper hole of depression. Don't ever be afraid to seek professional help.

It's the circle of life. We all enter this world and leave this world without knowing when that may be. My belief, it is all in universal timing – birth, death, and any loss we experience.

The death of a loved one or a pet is different to losing a career, relationship, or home. Losing someone close, a long-term relationship or a pet is a very deep grief from which we usually take longer to recover. With losing anything else, you still grieve but it may not be as deep. However, the feeling of loss can still be devastating.

Through my own experience, I have found that at times, I needed professional help through the early tough times. With the materialistic or professional losses, my body became sick up to a month until I learnt to accept, work through the process, and let go with the help of natural therapies.

Some of these experiences became massive turning points in my life, so I thank my lessons of grief as I learnt new ways of looking and dealing with loss to assist moving forward.

I still feel loss or grief when it happens, but I move into

more spiritual work now and find understanding and peace for me, which then allows me to support others in dealing with their grief.

Reflect on the good of the person, their life, or the situation that created the loss. Accepting that it was their time for whatever reason is difficult, but it is not ours to question, as hard as that can be.

This may sound like it was all easy, but I went through hell with grief and loss before I discovered the spiritual path that led me to greater acceptance and peace around death.

I still feel the sadness, tears, and loss but I now move through it more easily and with acceptance because I know everyone I have lost is now sending me love and guidance from above. The other losses in my life have set me on my purpose and path to a better way of looking at and living my life.

Find comfort in having something that reminds you of your loved one you can look at, wear, or create a small garden area for new growth and reflect on the love and memories. I have a beautiful framed photo of a stunning kookaburra on my wall reminding me of my father who died suddenly at 42 years old – he did the best kookaburra calls when we were kids. My favourite auntie's special painting (my dad's sister) hangs on another wall. These special pieces bring me great comfort, love, and memories.

Be kind, and nurture yourself during these times, especially if you are supporting others. Give yourself time and space.

Be patient, it will ease.

Here are a few reflection pieces that have assisted me during times of loss, the first of which I wrote myself after finding my way through grief.

The Passing

by Sharon Cairns

Birth is a miracle, and joy the beginning of a brand-new life!

Death is a mystery to us humans and nothing can ever prepare us for it.

How can we be prepared to lose someone or something we love even though we know, deep down, our lives and those we love and care for will come to an end. But when is the unknown?

We can prepare personal papers and share our wishes to our families. However, absolutely nothing prepares us for the emotions of loss and emptiness (the hole) we feel at that moment when our loved one takes their last breath.

The feelings of loss – denial, anger, loneliness and sadness, will flow through us in any order, with varying depths and forms. There is no right or wrong to how each one of us feels and for how long.

We struggle with the why, why, why... all those unanswered questions, especially if the person is young or taken from us suddenly. Old age, they have had their life, we understand and come to terms with it quicker.

Those who are still young, accidents, trauma, terminal

illness or the ones who have chosen to leave this life of their own free will. These tortured souls are in a pain and deep, deep sadness, truly believing the world is a better place without them. We are unable to relate to the depths that drives someone to suicide and it is the biggest 'Why?'.

Through my own personal experiences, it is truly difficult. The more we try to let go of the Why's, work through the grief with support and come to some understanding it is the 'Circle of Life'. A time of truly letting go. 'The Passing' from one world to another – the mystery we don't understand as humans, the more our grief will ease.

Allow yourself to fully grieve, release the sadness and loss, seek professional assistance, don't try and carry this on your own, draw on those offering their love and support.

Men need to be particularly conscious of this or any men you may know as they tend to say "I'm ok" then bottle it up inside – it's really good and important for men and boys to cry too!

Be very aware of children and their grief as well. It's ok and healthy to grieve – it's a deep emotion and talking it through is good medicine. Be patient, it's different for all of us, allow yourself time, be kind to yourself during the process and lean on those who truly love and care enough to support you.

Experiencing grief means we have truly loved someone or something, we never lose the love – it exists in us always. Eventually, all the emotions attached to grief soften, the numbness leaves us and we can allow ourselves to feel love, joy and peace again. Holding their memories in our hearts and lives, we begin to heal.

Life is for the living and that's what our lost loved ones would want for us, to keep living and loving life in their memory.

The Train

by John McDonald

At birth, we boarded the train and met our parents, and we believe they will always travel by our side. As time goes by, other people will board the train and they will be significant such as siblings, friends, children, and even the love of your life.

However, at some station, our parents will step down from the train, leaving us on this journey alone. Others will step down over time and leave a permanent vacuum. Some, however, will go unnoticed; that we don't even realise they vacated their seat.

This train ride will be full of joy, sorrow, fantasy, expectations, hellos, goodbyes, and farewells. Success consists of having a good relationship with all passengers, requiring that we give the best of ourselves.

The mystery to everyone is: we do not know at which station we will step down. So we must live in the best way, love, forgive, and offer the best of who we are. It is important to do this because when the time comes for us to step down and leave our seat empty, we should leave behind beautiful memories for those who will continue to travel on the train of life.

ACTION

PRACTISE BEING CALM,
HOLD LOVE IN YOUR HEART,
AND BE KIND TO YOURSELF
AND OTHERS!

Use breath-work – breathe in from the lower belly, feel the emotion, and release when you exhale. Really let it go. Yes, use sound as well like 'aaaaah', as loud as you like or cry it out! Repeat as often as you need.

There is also grief yoga, which I found helped me. It's a process of breathing, releasing stored emotions and then planting new seeds of life like a new garden. (Google Paul Denniston – Grief Yoga and David Kessler – Grief.com)

Supporting Others

If you are a support person for someone grieving don't be afraid to ask them "How are you feeling today?" It gives them the opportunity to open up and talk, don't just accept "I'm ok" as an answer. Say, "I know you're feeling vulnerable, sad, angry, lonely; I'm here to listen and offer any support I can."

Make contact with them daily, even just a 'Thinking of you' text message, especially needed after all the formalities are over and others go back to their lives and routines. People drop off in the early days of grieving as they often don't know how to deal with or what to say anymore.

The days, weeks and months after the formalities is a

really important time to support someone. Assisting them to gain understanding, perspective and guide them through the changes of creating a new life that will never be the same as before. Show them there is hope and opportunities to move forward.

As the support person you need to truly let them talk, express their emotions without judgement, really listen and stay present during the conversation. Even if they are repeating the same things, be patient with them. If you feel they need professional guidance/support, don't be afraid to suggest it. Attend with them if they need you, even just the first session or just be waiting outside so they can debrief if needed.

Be brave and honest enough to say to them:

"I can't remove or change the pain and grief you are feeling, unfortunately it is the process of grief. However, I am here to hold your hand and support you through the pain until you feel stronger."

- Daily text message or phone call. Just check in on them and reassure them you are there for them – keep it brief but listen.

- Once a week meet them for a meal or walk, talk and coffee, meet in a different place each time to give them variety. If walking doesn't suit them maybe a lovely drive and coffee – allow them to talk and cry it out. Once you feel they are coping better emotionally, change it to once a fortnight then once month, this gradually gives them the strength to cope and move forward.

- Assist them to find interests they would enjoy to fill

the gap of loss but don't push them into activities you think suit them, just keep it as suggestions for them to think about while allowing them to choose their new pathway.

- A Bucket List of things they might like to do in the future. Important to offer assistance with paperwork, clearing belongings etc., or even just keeping them company at legal or medical appointments until they feel sorted. Be aware of when to step back, don't push too much.

Don't smother them, give them space and allow them the power to find their way!

CHAPTER 23

PEACE

These quotes say it perfectly. Once you start living your life well, you will gain peace!

"Peace. It does not mean to be in a place where there is no trouble, noise, or hard work. It means to be in the midst of those things and still be calm in your heart."

~Lady Gaga

"Peace is not just the absence of conflict; peace is the creation of an environment where all can flourish."

~Nelson Mandela

CHAPTER 24

CREATING FLOW

Manage your life a little more, and I don't mean every single thing in a full-on, micro-managed, spreadsheet kind of way. Try not to be overly structured and allow for flexibility and fun to enjoy your life!

The aim is to organise and manage your life more simply to ease anxiety, and stress, and feel less burdened so your life and world will flow more easily.

Believing in yourself, your pathway, and trusting the flow of life brings lightness.

Letting go is also part of creating flow. So if there is an area in your life that challenges you or creates stress, the 'art of letting go' or surrendering, creates more flow!

Being in the flow should feel effortless.

When you're holding onto anger, you have less room for love.

When you're holding onto resentment, you have less room for happiness.

When you're holding onto fear, you have less room for creativity.

It feels sooooo good to just LET GO!

ACTION

Research meditation apps that will help you understand how to let go and surrender. The art of not being attached to the outcomes is a difficult but great thing to master.

MY FAVOURITES APPS

- Calm – lots varied subjects to meditate on and sleep stories.

- Headspace – anxiety, depression.

- Smiling Minds.

- Deepak Chopra and Oprah: 21-day meditations

- Oprah on 'Surrendering'.

- Have fun and put it into practise daily if possible – just 10 minutes a day is achievable, and great results gained.

- Use the guidelines on the following pages to get you started.

Everyone's daily lives are different so adjust to suit your life – let your life move and flow like the tides of the ocean and... Enjoy the benefits of your daily routines!

"If you are acting like a sheep, do not blame the shepherd. You cannot herd lions – so wake up and roar."

~Apache proverb

CHAPTER 25

DAILY MORNING ROUTINE

- Rise 15 minutes earlier than usual.

- Refrain from social media until after stretching, eating, and preparing for your day – the world can wait!

- Sip warm water with sliced lemon – it wakes the body up and assists in digestion.

- Stretch, meditate, or just walk outside in nature for a few minutes.

- Eat a healthy breakfast because it's the most important meal of the day – carbs and protein combined create energy.

- Exercise (I personally need fruit or a smoothie before exercise).

- Shower – finish with a cold-blast of water all over your body because this stimulates and energises your whole system. Work it up and down your spine (stimulates the central nervous system) say, "every cell in my body is healthy and full of energy to meet all my needs today."

- While drying off, look in the mirror and say, "I love my body, and I love me."

- Moisturise your body lightly (my favourite at the moment is organic apricot oil from the health food shop).

- Dress into something that makes U feel good and that suits your daily lifestyle.

- Makeup is a choice – some days we like to wear it and others not at all.

- Perfume is also a choice to wear or not to wear, whichever suits U.

- Write a to-do list for the day – even just one or two things you need to complete so you don't overwhelm yourself.

- Lessen your time on social media – only check in during your breaks and not while walking around the streets or driving. Instead, put your head up, look where you're going, keep your eye on the horizon and take in the environment. Listen to those around you, especially your children, and communicate personally.

- Be kind to yourself and to others.

- Smile not because you feel you have to or someone has told U to. Smile for yourself, who U are and how U feel – a true genuine smile comes from within.

Mindset – gratitude for the day, your life, and U – Enjoy!

CHAPTER 26

DAILY EVENING ROUTINE

- On your way home, just let go of work/school plus any negative stuff from the day and prepare your mind for home.

- Begin a calmer mindset before you walk through the door at home.

- This can be hard if you're a busy mum or dad but perhaps some calming music can help you and others to settle before arriving home.

- Arrive home and kick off those shoes and walk barefoot for a while.

- Aromatherapy diffuser with de-stress oil in main living area/kitchen.

- Walk or exercise if this fits your routine in the evening or just sit for five minutes outside is nice. Breathe and gather your thoughts.

- Have the children run around outside for a while, join them if you wish. Enjoy the fresh air and the freedom!

- Supervise homework and feed or walk pets, but don't forget to delegate and share the load.

- Prepare a delicious, simple, and healthy dinner.

- Sit down together. It may be hard with a busy family but try at least a few nights a week. Make sure that you don't use phones and other devices and the TV is turned off. Watch the news later.

- Talk and ask those who share your table how their day was. Ask about the worst thing that happened and then the best part of their day. Give everyone time and space to share their day and offer support for any issues or celebrate their success.

- Share the tasks of cleaning up and preparing the food, clothes, bags, and anything else needed for the following day, so that your day starts with more flow and less chaos – delegate.

- Have a dedicated sleep/charging area for all devices in your home two hours before bed. This includes parents as well – set the example.

- There may be homework and work projects needed to be completed but try and schedule this earlier in the evening so you can disconnect and turn off devices 1-2 hours before bed. Read to your children from a real book.

- Our brains are wired and working hard all day so let it rest, recover, and recharge just like our computers.

- Chill out with your favourite TV show and a nurturing warm drink.

- Curl up and turn the pages of a real book in bed just for U!

- Incorporate bedtime rituals for all – going to bed at the same time most nights of the week signals to our body that it's time to rest and recover!

- Read, meditate, do yoga stretches for sleep, and listen to calming music. If you have trouble nodding off maybe a natural sleep supplement will help.

- Refrain from using devices in the bedroom, especially for the children – the devices all go to the sleep station. If you're concerned about your alarm, buy a small bedside clock for everyone just like we used to use, or there are bedside lamps now with digital clocks built in.

- Bedtime bath or shower in the evening is a personal choice OR a warm footbath for your feet with Magnesium flakes and a few drops of a calming oil blend is a nice option.

- Keep heating to a minimum and only if needed in bedrooms. No electric blankets, wear warm pjs and warm flannelette sheets instead, and use a warm wheatbag if needed.

- If you're having trouble settling-in or sleeping, aromatherapy is helpful. Find a nice sleep blend in an aromatherapy diffuser with a timer OR just use one drop of lavender, sleep blend oil and rub onto the bottom of your feet at night – if no skin allergies to the oils.

- Magnesium oil is also very relaxing when rubbed onto the bottom of your feet when going to bed. Great for all ages.

Allow your body to rest, relax, recover, and recharge every night!

CHAPTER 27

WEEKLY

Get sorted and organised for the week ahead. A bit of effort makes life flow a lot more easily!

- Food shop once a week. How wonderful is online shopping and deliveries, which is just perfect for our busy lives.

- Set aside some time once a week to sit down and plan. The more you do this, the easier it becomes.

- Have a board or list in the kitchen and ask everyone in the household to write down when something runs out. Then your shopping list is partly done!

- Meal plan – write down a few dinner ideas for the next five days. See if you can make something last two nights in a row. Slow cookers are a great example! At the end of the week, just use all the remaining fresh veggies and make a stir fry or soup. You can add rice, pulses or pasta to bulk it up if needed. Meat-free, healthy, and easy! Enjoy one night a week off cooking.

- Lunches – think about what to make for lunch in the next five days, including fruits and snacks like nuts and yoghurt. Boil eggs and keep them in the fridge, and they can be a great little nutritional bomb for lunch!

- Breakfast – prepare, even if it's a smoothie, fruit, cereal, toast, or a Sunday cook-up!

- Healthy snacks – fruit, dips, nuts, cheese, and biscuits for the hungries before dinner! Pre-cut carrots, celery, and cucumber – delegate this job early in the week.

- Write your shopping list for the week and when all ingredients are there, you don't have to worry. No racing minds and no stressful visits to the supermarket on the way home – nothing else to worry about at the end of your busy day!

Of course if you're solo, a couple, or have a busy family life, consider one of the online delivery services to bring in fresh food boxes with all you need for the week. There are good, organic, pre-made options in Melbourne: Dynamic Organic Meals, Hello Fresh etc. There are so many choices available, so just find what suits you and your budget, then sit down, place your order, and it's done. Out of your mind and off the to-do list!

It takes a bit of effort to start creating a system once a week, along with the sorting. However, the rest of the week will flow, and you will have less stress and more time once you arrive home. Also, weekly shopping should work out more economical than buying daily.

This also flows over to organising clothes for the week ahead – work, sports, etc.

All this saves time, money, and stress.

WEEKENDS

Gotta love weekends!

*Permission to let loose,
have fun, and relax!*

FOLLOW SOME OF YOUR DAILY RITUALS, BUT THIS IS THE TIME TO ENJOY ALL THOSE THINGS YOU REALLY LOVE!

- Break loose from the routines – of course, there's the laundry and cleaning, but you can put on some upbeat music, dance, and sing through it! Also, don't forget to delegate.

- Enjoy walks or bike rides along the beach, park, or countryside. Have coffee or ice cream along the way.

- Catch up with friends and family – spend time with those you love and who make you laugh, share a simple meal together.

- Sleep in a little.

- Night off cooking – eat out or in with takeaway.

- Indulge with having ice cream or chocolate, just as

long as it's not too much.

- Relax with a glass of wine, beer, or a non-alcoholic cocktail.

- Take a long warm bath with a book and glass of wine.

- Watch movies. Even lose yourself in kids' movies – it's fun!

- Go outside and enjoy gardening, kick a ball with kids or play with your pets. Breathe in the fresh air and the environment or just sit and listen to the birds or nature to ground yourself.

- Enjoy a big, cook-up Sunday breaky or brunch and have everyone stay in their pjs.

- Lessen social media – try one day or morning without it, and that includes everyone!

It's not always ideal to have the whole weekend like this but make a ritual so that at least one of your days on a weekend is a free, easy, let-loose kind of day!

Let loose, enjoy your life, and have a great weekend!

CHAPTER 28

MONTHLY

Life throws us lots of 'left fields', which can divert any of us off our path, so check your progress each month – anything out of balance? Diarise a date with yourself each month to keep you moving forward and finding balance.

· Do I need to delegate more?

· Motivate or focus more?

· Do my body and my mind feel that I need some time-out, even just for a day?

· Am I feeling stressed, anxious or overwhelmed?

· Am I eating and exercising well?

· Am I getting enough sound sleep?

· How's my budget tracking this month? Have I overspent?

· Have I started my 'fun fund' coin jar?

· Do I need to change the way I am thinking about some issues or people in my life? Personal or career?

Once a month, spend just a little time reflecting, adjusting, and bringing balance back into your life. Remember that it is a constant juggling act – no blame, shame or punishing yourself. Just do your best!

Nothing happens without action!

CHAPTER 30

YEARLY - REFLECTION ACTIVITY

Make an appointment with U in your diary

- End each year by setting aside some quiet time after the Christmas chaos.

- Write out a reflection list of everything you have achieved or been proud of in the past year, including the lessons you have learnt.

- Issues or problems – how you handled and solved them, what the outcome was, and if faced with this again, how you could improve your attitude and outcome. Maybe celebrate how well you handled it!

They don't have to be big business deals:

- Maybe you sorted a better daily routine.

- Gave up smoking or sugar.

- Lost a few kilos.

- Exercised more.

- Made a few new choices and changes.

- De-cluttered.

- Less social media.

- Took a few breaks or finally had a holiday.

- Been kinder to yourself and others.

- Feeling less stressed, healthier and more balanced.

Read over it and feel proud and good about U!

Note any improvements you could make in the New Year.

Family and partners can join in this ritual – a morning or afternoon to reflect and celebrate U!

This is self-praise, which builds our self-worth and self-love.

Keep the list and pin it up somewhere so you can reflect often on your success!

Then the New Year

For the New Year, write a list of things you would like to aim for and what action you can do to support achieving them.

Again, it doesn't have to be a huge, overwhelming list. It can be as simple as one thing or one change a month. Remember to make it achievable, not overwhelming!

Add a quote that you relate to that keeps you motivated. Write in a different colour a few words that express how you would like to feel in the coming year, such as happiness, gratitude, peace, contentment, harmony, healthy, balanced, joy, or love. You can string a few together but keep it simple – these are your personal power words for the year!

Read over and pin up with your previous year's reflection list and have fun with it. Use highlight pens or draw pictures around it.

HAVE FUN!

CHAPTER 31

MY PHILOSOPHY ON LIFE

- Keep everything simple. Life is simple. It's humans and technology that complicate it.

- Love U every day! Celebrate, respect and honour your uniqueness for who you are, you truly count and make a difference by how far you have come and your own special gifts.

- Try and aim for more balance in every area of your daily life.

- Eat and exercise for your well-being. Try eating and moving with the seasons.

- Be the best U can be each day. That may vary day-to-day but that's ok as long as it's no one else's version. Work towards it one step at a time.

- Clear the clutter as often as needed in all areas of your life.

- Stay away from negative/draining people, issues, and drama.

- Put the past behind U. Work on the NOW and moving forward.

- U have the choice each day to start a new future.

- Gratitude every day, even for just one thing. Focus on what you have, not what you don't.

- Kindness – practise this daily. One random act of kindness, even if it's just a smile or hello to someone you don't know. Simple things that makes someone else's day.

- Tomorrow is a new day.

- Keep calm and breathe.

- Be happy – whatever that is to U! Find your happy place.

- Love, hug, and spend time with those who love U and lift your energy.

- Enjoy this one, amazing life U have been given.

*"Don't save anything for a special occasion.
Being alive is the special occasion."*

~Anonymous

CHAPTER 32

REFLECTION
- ACTION

- Now, re-look at yourself in the mirror. How do you feel about U?

- Write a list of how U now see yourself overall – mind, body, happiness, changes, and balance. How is your life now after making some changes? How are you feeling?

- Ask that same person who wrote how they saw you at the start of this journey, to write how they see you now and the changes they have noticed in U.

- Compare both letters and celebrate!

Acknowledge how far U have come
and all that U have learned.
Recognise how much U have given
and how much U have received.

I LOVE myself for being ME!

Appreciate and Celebrate U
- Do a Happy Dance !

The more you work on U, the more peace and freedom will be yours. I wish you well in finding more Balance, Peace, Joy, Health and Happiness in your life.

"The privilege of a lifetime is being who U are."

~Joseph Campbell

BEST OF ALL, ENJOY AND CELEBRATE BEING THE BEST U

AND

LIVE YOUR LIFE WELL EVERY DAY!

SENDING YOU
MUCH LOVE
AND
INSPIRATION

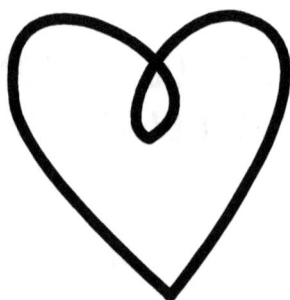

Sharon

Kinesiologist, Qest4 Bioresonance Practitioner,
Advanced PSYCH-K® Facilitator, Qigong Facilitator,
author of *Wellness with the Seasons*

sharoncairnsrye@gmail.com

www.thriveandshinehealth.com.au

RESOURCES MYSELF, MY FAMILY, FRIENDS AND CLIENTS HAVE PERSONALLY FOUND HELPFUL

- *Wellness with the Seasons* author Sharon Cairns.
- Apps – Calm, Tapping Solution, Headspace, Smiling Minds.
- Lee Harris *Monthly Energy Updates* You Tube and his many Online Courses.
- Mel Robbins *The Let Them Theory* and her many Podcasts
- Deepak and Oprah 21-day meditations.
- Align and Attract – Kerry Rowett alignandattract.com.
- Grief Yoga – Paul Denniston, Grief.com – David Kessler.
- Tony Robbins YouTube on relationships.
- Finance Books: Scott Pape – *The Barefoot Investor* and *The Barefoot Investor for Families*. David Bach – *The Latte Factor, Start Late Finish Rich* and many other interesting titles.
- The Aussie pre-prepared food deliveries – Dynamics Organic and Hello Fresh both deliver to your door.

ACKNOWLEDGEMENTS

To family, friends and special sisterhood, my wonderful clients, past employers, staff, teachers, mentors, trainers, my natural health practitioners and doctors who keep me well. Authors of the many books I have read, healers, personal relationships, and everyone who has passed through my life – thank you for the lessons you have contributed, by supporting and helping me grow into who I am – *Me!*

My original writing mentor and author, June Loves – without meeting you first, this book would never have been written.

My friend and associate, Sue Boal – you have kept me well, motivated, inspired, on track and pushed me through my sabotage barriers, which gave me the confidence to believe in myself!

My dear friend Maggie for your proofreading, love, support and encouragement – thank you.

Thank you to my publishing consultant, Julie Postance – IInspire Media and her team – Sophie White, designer and layout artist; and editor, Amanda J Spedding – for their professional guidance and holding my hand through the process of a first-time author. It's been an awesome experience, ladies, regardless of the speed bumps along the way. You have all kept me inspired!

ABOUT THE AUTHOR

Sharon Cairns is a natural health practitioner running her own Natural Health Studio, *Thrive and Shine Health.*

Sharon is a qualified and experienced Kinesiologist and Qest 4 Bioresonance Practitioner, who works very holistically; pysch-k facilitator, massage therapist, Qigong (chi-gong) facilitator, has a TAA training qualification and many other natural health modalities gained over many years. Passionate about health, life, and guiding others, Sharon puts the focus particularly on women to achieve a more balanced, stress-free life.

She is a loving, dedicated and proud mum to 3 amazing sons, mother-in-law and beach Nanna to their ever extending families of beautiful children. Bringing up an all-male household has been a challenge, but given her experience and many life lessons, it has resulted in much love and joy in her life!

Her personal journey from ill health many years before has led her to become well through personal growth, natural therapy, education, and study. After many years, she has finally found her purpose and path, which has and continues to give her balance, joy, happiness and peace with life!

In her book, Sharon shares her story drawn from her own life experience, professional knowledge, wisdom, and passion for health and balance in life gained over many years. This is an easy read full of simple tips, knowledge, and guidance, assisting you to be *"The Best U"* can be by understanding, accepting, loving, and discovering who **you really** are and no one else's version. The outcome is for you to gain better health, happiness, balance, peace, and flow to make a difference in your everyday life!

Sharon lives and works in a beautiful coastal town in Melbourne, Victoria.

Sometimes the smallest changes in your life can have the greatest impact.